# PTSD COMPASS

# PTSD Compass

## NAVIGATE TRAUMA TO TRIUMPH AND RENEW YOUR LIFE

Pantea Kalhor

Acechoice Inc.

# *Contents*

# PTSD Compass

How to Recover from PTSD and Navigate Trauma to Triumph
Through Mind-Body Connection

Pantea Kalhor
Nancy Nance, Roseline Salazar, Maricelly Ramos, Richard Morden,
Linda Hayes Cooper
Edited by Angela Curtis

ACECHOICE
PUBLISHING &
BRANDING

# Copyright

PTSD Compass



ISBN-13: 978-1-7780351-2-8



http://acechoiceidea.com
AceChoice Publishing and Branding

# Claim Your Freebies

Join the summit email list and claim your freebies and complementary consultation from our authors and speakers.

https://panteakalhor.com/ptsd-summit-oct-2021/

# Keep in Touch

Do you have a story to share and to see yourself as a published author? Connect with me here:

http://acechoiceidea.com

Are you a PTSD warrior and would like to have some inspiration or to learn about mind-body connection healing? Follow the link below:

https://panteakalhor.com/ptsd-summit-oct-2021/

You can also subscribe to my channel to get the latest interviews:

https://www.youtube.com/PanteaKalhorTransitionChannel

Podcast:

https://panteakalhor.libsyn.com/

Keep in touch by visiting my Facebook and Instagram pages:

Facebook, Instagram: @panteakalhorcoach

# This Book is Dedicated to

**My husband,** my best friend, and love of my life. His patience through this entire process and his kind support kept me inspired to accomplish my mission of sharing stories of hope and healing.

**My Parents,** my anchors, my shelter, and my safety. I was so blessed to have them over in Canada during my summit and book launch.

**My beautiful daughter** who let me be her mother and feel the real depth of motherhood. My world totally changed by her birth. She even changed my career path and my life's purpose.

**My authors and contributors** who believed in me and supported me in participating my summits and reading and my books.

**My readers,** PTSD Survivors who read my book and support me by watching my podcast interviews. Through all interviews with PTSD coaches, healers, doctors, and holistic medicine practitioners, I learned that life is so beautiful and worthy to live. There is always hope, even in a dark tunnel when your eyes are blind, and you can't navigate to a brighter path. I found hope after trauma, after war, loss, immigration, violence, and infertility.

*Life is worth living.*

Pantea Kalhor

Oct 20th 2021

# Other Books by Pantea Kalhor

Rules of Change for the Better: Real Stories and Your Guide to Tune-Up Your Mood and Transform Your Life to Reach Your Biggest Dreams

https://www.amazon.com/dp/B07MKZ91R1

Naturally Conceived: How to Get Pregnant, Explain Unexplained Infertility and Prevent Miscarriages by Unleashing Your Reproductive Power Even Over 40!

https://www.amazon.com/dp/1999545842

# FOREWORD Dr Defne Nayman MD Antiaging, Functional, and Metabolic Medicine Expert, International Speaker, Author

As an emergency medicine physician for many years, I have experienced a variety of traumatic events, and in my personal life, I have endured my fair share of traumatic experiences. I grasp how PTSD (Post-Traumatic Stress Disorder) affects souls as well as the mind and body.

We find our own unique ways to heal from our traumatic experiences, and we start looking at the events from a different perspective with a fresh set of eyes. I like the embodiment of what Tony Robbins says: "Blame the events for who we became, who we are now."

Hearteningly, I met Pantea through an influential mentorship program, and I am an avid admirer of her tireless work in bringing experts together to explore topics relevant to many of us. She is raising awareness and educating people by bringing exclusively selected experts with their wisdom to the table.

Listening to the PTSD self-healing summit was deeply emotional and equally uplifting. Standing ovation to all the writers in the book who are fearlessly forthcoming about their most terrifying memories and sharing their ways out of their deepest, darkest times.

# FOREWORD By Erin Chandler Intuitive Healer, Psychic Medium, and Author

Throughout our lives, we often meet with trauma, tragedy, loss, and negative experiences that can alter our world as we know it. It is because of these experiences that we struggle in the darkness of those traumas and the aftershocks that change our perception of our lives from that point on. I have been on that journey, like many. After the death of my youngest daughter, storytelling became a significant part of my healing process. Spirituality I came to believe that we can heal ourselves with various tools and the support of community.

As a psychic, medium, and intuitive healer, working with many suffering from trauma and grief, I found when we delve into the expansive realm of possibility, into the unknown, we can learn how to talk about our deepest wounds. In a safe community, we can learn to understand our journey and embrace the profound, and life changing healing process that takes place.

Despite the horrors, traumas, and negative experiences we have, they can ultimately lead us to positive and compassionate people that understand us. Those who have been where we are. Those who have overcome and transcended their traumas and their aftereffects.

Pantea Kalhor is one of those people. We met through our mutual desire to help others find alternative ways to heal themselves from the aftershocks, the residue of trauma, and the tragedy that creates PTSD. We had an instant connection, recognizing that more people need to speak up and out about their experiences after trauma. Not just how to heal PTSD, but to dig deep and analyze our emotions. To learn how to live with the consequences and find healing.

Pantea is a soul warrior, driven by her desire to serve others, both by her own work in healing infertility and her experience of being held at knifepoint. She found a way to overcome these traumatic experiences and recognized that other people from many walks of life and experiences, have also found ways to heal themselves from PTSD trauma.

Her heartfelt dedication to helping others overcome trauma is the foundation of the PTSD Summit. Founded by Pantea, it is a collaboration of multiple modalities, and stories from those who have traversed the dark landscape of PTSD. This summit created a space for healing for all who attended, even the warriors as they shared their testimonies and the tools they use.

This book results from that PTSD Summit. It's a compilation of all their incredible stories—the heartbreak of trauma, their healing journey, how they built resilience and found answers. These inspiring warriors, speak about how they took their power back and overcame all that held them down. Pantea has woven each of these moving accounts together for those who are struggling with the aftereffects of trauma, loss, and PTSD.

Each story here will touch your heart and inspire you to find your own healing path, to thrive despite of the trauma, to refuse to let trauma run this show called life, and to take back your power through these different modalities of healing. Everyone is an intuitive – including YOU!

Thank you for shining a light for those still on the healing path, Pantea!

Erin E Chandler[1]

# Editorial Note

PTSD was a term mainly associated with the armed and emergency services. But with traumatic events occurring around the world, it's increasing the prevalence of the condition throughout the general population. With all the fear and restrictions being enforced at present, there is a critical need for greater public awareness about this life-altering condition.

If you have been diagnosed, or think you may have PTSD, I want to encourage you to read this book. No matter where you are on the path to recovery, inside these pages you'll find advice and the motivation to start your healing journey. Pantea has collaborated with a group of experts, who like her, have all experienced PTSD and found ways to recover. A valuable resource, a light of hope that shines into the darkness and illuminates the path to healing.

I'm a survivor of an abusive marriage, numerous car accidents, and death experiences. (I didn't enjoy dying, so I've decided, I'm not doing that again!). I was diagnosed as having the highest level on the PTSD scale. I wasn't surprised. What did amaze me was being told traumatic events compound over a lifetime. That those like me, who suffered at the hand of an abuser, such as rape and physical assault, suffered more damage than those living through natural disasters or freak accidents.

I have also learned first-hand that the discrimination and prejudice of the ill-informed can feel worse than the illness itself and exacerbate the symptoms.

As someone who has experienced all levels of this disorder, the most remarkable breakthrough came when I read about recent studies made by neuropathologists. They stated PTSD causes both brain and physical damage. Sadly, it took a psychiatrist to tell me that this could be measured and confirmed before I felt less ashamed, felt more accepting of myself and my symptoms.

With further research, I discovered PTSD increases cortisol and norepinephrine levels. It has a detrimental effect on the Amygdala, which is responsible for emotions, instincts, memory, and survival. It gathers information to determine any threats and, if it detects danger, it becomes hyperactive.

It's taken time, but with a lot of work, patience, and self-care, I have found peace and now, I rarely get PTSD symptoms. If I do, I know how to handle the triggers, so the experience is brief.

If you've suffered from persisting symptoms that come and go, or are re-activated by reminders of the traumatic event, keep reading. The experts' effective solutions and strategies can help you heal and live your best life. I've experienced remarkable results using these same treatments. My life is forever changed. There is hope for you. Your internal scars and physical symptoms will heal. You can recover. You are not alone.

I am an overcomer! You can be one too!

Read on Dear Warrior. Your freedom is near.

Angela Curtis, Best-Selling Author/Lecturer

# Praise for PTSD Compass

**Fabulous Stories of Hope and Healing**

Seventy percent of adults in the United States have experienced some type of a traumatic event at least once in their lifetimes. Fortunately, as Pantea Kalhor illustrates in this powerful book, there is life after trauma.

The stories that Kalhor shares - from her own harrowing experience of being robbed to tales of losing children and spouses - will make you realize you are not alone. You'll also discover dozens of healing modalities that can help you cope with loss and move forward with your life. Some are obvious, like therapy and yoga. Others, like Gang Shui and aromatherapy, are surprising.

If you are struggling with PTSD or trauma, read this book and you'll be inspired and informed so you can heal.

**Experts share their PTSD stories and solutions**

This book contains a collection of personal stories as well as healing solutions from several experts. No matter what type of PTSD applies to you—grief, relationship abuse, first responder recovery, military abuse, childhood abuse, infertility, or domestic violence— there is something for everyone.

It is like Chicken Soup for the Soul for PTSD. Highly recommend for anyone who suffers from PTSD or works with people who suffer from PTSD.

**Phenomenal book of different author's experiences and their healing journey.**

This book is a need to read for those suffering from domestic violence and PTSD. These authors are from all walks of life, different backgrounds and professions, who share their experience and solutions to their healing journeys. Each story has a powerful message that helps empower and motivate one another. I truly believe this book will impact your lives positively.

**A great resource for those with PTSD and their families**

This is an excellent resource for people who have suffered - or who think they may be suffering - from Post-Traumatic Stress Disorder. Multiple authors offer multiple viewpoints and a myriad of experiences that are sure to speak to any individual in their personal situation.

Highly recommend!

**A welcome light during dark times**

*PTSD Compass* is a book that's time has come. Many people in the world are suffering not only from "pandemic fallout," but harboring deep, unhealed stress from all kinds of trauma. Those who have PTSD need to know they're not alone. They also need to know they can take their power back and create a better life for themselves. The stories in this book show all of that and much more. I highly recommend Pantea's compilation of many authors' experiences and wisdom. A welcome light during dark times.

**Great Resource**

Wow, there are so many resources and experts on healing from PTSD packed into this book! It was encouraging to hear their personal stories and see how many options there are for PTSD recovery. Definitely a valuable resource as you seek out tools for your own journey.

**Powerful and moving. The title says, "How to..." but this book doesn't tell, it shows.**

A well-structured book full of so many real examples of people who became who they are when they allowed themselves to heal from trauma. Trauma comes in many forms. This book is a blend of people from different backgrounds who share their stories of darkness, but the weight of this book's message centers around the light. The light which can be found beyond the trauma.

**Collection of Wisdom**

*PTSD Compass* has many beautiful stories of recovery from trauma. Open up the book, and on every page, you will find some inspiration and hope. If you are looking to overcome trauma, then *PTSD Compass* is the book for you!

**Source of Inspiration**

Stories of inspiration to help you or your loved ones overcome trauma. Such a valuable resource in these trying times.

# Disclaimer

"PTSD Compass" speakers and authors who have suffered from PTSD share the solutions they used on their journey to recovery. As a collective, we have given you a variety of valuable tools to help you on your own journey. But it's imperative you do your own research and seek advice before practicing any of the modalities enclosed.

The authors and publisher do not intend to diagnose, treat, cure, or prevent any condition or disease. Please consult with your own physician or healthcare specialist concerning the suggestions and recommendations made in this book.

This book is not intended as a substitute for consultation with a licensed healthcare practitioner, such as your physician. Before you begin any healthcare program, or change your lifestyle in any way, you should consult your physician or another licensed healthcare practitioner to choose the right tool.

PTSD Compass provides content related to physical and/or mental health issues. As such, use of this book implies your acceptance of this disclaimer.

# Introduction

If you scream, I'll kill you, said the shadow of death that darkened my shoulder. I felt the evil soul dig a knife into my belly in an attempt to steal what belonged to me. Not only my car, but my health, my courage, and my identity. This ruthless stranger was holding me captive while trying to cut through my seat belt.

My mind went crazy trying to make sense of it all. *Is this really happening to me? Am I awake? Or is this a horror movie?* His warning to remain silent validated my worst fears. This was real. I was just threatened with assassination all over a car. But no matter how many times he warned me to be silent, I couldn't do it. I could just let him kill me. He could have the car. I just wanted to keep my life.

Despite his threats, I took a deep breath and screamed with all the energy I had, praying I wouldn't be killed. I begged for someone to hear me. I wanted to be heard. I needed to stay alive. I still had so many dreams yet to fulfill.

My screams made him cut at the belt with more urgency and force. Within seconds, he'd cut his way through, but instead of stabbing me, he grabbed my arm and threw me out of my car. I continued to scream, asking for help. *Was anybody else out there? Could anyone hear my voice?* When I think back to that time even now, it's clear that when trauma hit, I felt like I'd been robbed.

**

Have you suffered from trauma? What has been stolen from you? Your childhood, your confidence, your trust, your youth, your femininity, your happiness? Or are you close to someone who is going on this journey, and you want to help?

It's terrifying to learn that within a few seconds, your entire life can change forever. An accident or traumatic incident can leave its footprints on the cells of your body cells, in the depths of your heart and in the hidden places of your memory.

Sometimes the trauma is a sequence of overwhelming events which reshapes your identity and changes your core beliefs long term. For example, being raised in a dysfunctional family, living the horror of an abusive relationship, suffering from abandonment, loss, or any type of negative experience in your life, they all alter you.

I assumed everything was fine until I saw, heard, smelt, tasted, or touched something that brought it all back. All the hidden memories and flashbacks to where I suffered that trauma.

The reminder of my accident followed me for years. I had to deal with my unprocessed trauma on a continual basis. These triggers raised feelings of fear. Even though I knew I was no long being followed, that I was not about to be murdered, the terror of that night haunted me.

"I am fine," I told myself over and over. But was I truly fine? It took me a few years to be honest with myself. It was time to find a way to start over. I was determined to shift my mindset, retrain my brain, and rebuild my life again. I did not want to live in fear anymore. I was done with its effects and its confinement.

## Why Did I Write This Book?

To advocate for mental health and Post-Traumatic Stress Disorder, I wrote and published my first book, *Rules of Change for the Better*[2]. I launched it in December of 2018 and shared my post-trauma recovery journey with the world.

My journey didn't stop there. I had to recover from another trauma. The trauma of infertility. So, I wrote and published my second book *Naturally Conceived*[3], in collaboration with 22 fertility experts and holistic practitioners. After which I became a fertility coach, an advocate, and certified in Post-Traumatic Stress Disorder and Cognitive Behavioral Therapy. I wanted to help women who struggle with fertility issues or have lost their babies in recurrent miscarriages. I wanted to give them hope.

June 2021, in mental health awareness month, I created the PTSD Self-Healing Summit and converted it to "PTSD Compass" book.

I gathered top experts from around the world in different areas of "Post Traumatic Stress Disorder" treatment, such as grief and loss, miscarriages, domestic violence, and abusive relationships.

I learned how mind-body connection can improve the healing process; no matter if you suffer from suicidal thoughts, combat PTSD, transgenerational PTSD, or first responders' PTSD. I hope suggested modalities and alternative healing approaches can bring hope and support to all who have lost their loved ones. Especially during the global pandemic.

If you're isolated from your family and friends, or have battled with mental or physical health, this book is for you. I believe that the pages within can give you hope, open new windows to your future, and enable you to learn the coping mechanisms so you can live your best life.

Living for 47-years in three different countries has brought a lot of challenges for me. I've learned to adapt to them. No matter what you have suffered, or how long ago it happened, I believe there is hope for you if you try these solutions which have been experienced and tested by our experts.

You can learn more about my life's challenges in my first book: *Rules of Change for the Better*[4].

This book is about how I and many others have gone through different stages of PTSD. How we've learned how to cope with sudden changes, and manage the transition after trauma, and how to create desired and sustainable adjustments to improve your lives in the best possible way.

We are all guided by intuition. The pandemic showed us how one tiny virus could change the structure of the entire world. That proved how we are all connected. If you are reading this book, your intuition has guided you here. This is not an accident! You have taken the first step in transforming your life. Inside this book, we all share real-life events to show you there is a life after trauma.

Even if we have lost our loved ones, or we are in an abusive relationship purely for the sake of protecting our kids, we are still living and thriving. If you've had to leave your family to get away from violence, or you're stuck in a war zone, been assaulted, or even lost your home, you are not alone.

If you are determined to rebuild your life, heal from trauma, and invite joy to fill your life again, then you are in the right place. This book is a gift from us to you. Welcome to the beginning of your new life.

# PTSD Self-Healing Summit, Part 1

I recorded the PTSD Self-Healing Summit on June 23-June 24, 2021.

Day 1 of the Summit focused on grief-recovery, Miscarriage and Prenatal Trauma, domestic violence, and abusive relationships.

https://youtu.be/dwB0T_rl0Qg

Day 2 of the Summit was about mind-body connection and how PTSD can affect our overall health.

https://youtu.be/j5PwnyYbkio

Part 1 explains recorded videos. It clarifies the topics we discussed at the summit.

# CHAPTER 1: Grief Recovery

A heavy feeling weighed in my stomach, yet I hadn't been able to eat properly since morning. I could hear my mother and aunts mourning downstairs. I was sitting with my cousins at my late aunt's funeral, grieving and reviewing her memories. It was hard to believe we had lost such a beautiful lady, whose biggest wish was to see her daughter go to school. Before she got married, she joined us on most of my family trips. She and I shared a deep bond.

She fought with cancer for over five years. In the fifth year, the cancer spread viciously all over her body. My mother brought her home so she could take care of her. She stayed with us for a year. Her husband brought her daughter to our place sometimes and I remember one night how tightly she hugged her and sang to her for hours until they both fell asleep.

When I checked on her to cover her with a blanket, her tears were still rolling down her cheeks from the corner of her eyes. She had her daughter wrapped tightly in her arms and held her daughter's hands in hers. Now, years later, when I think back to those days, I look at my beautiful 3-year-old daughter and I understand the bond she had with her child, and the secret intensity behind the melancholy farewell song.

The fear of leaving your baby in this unpredictable world is indescribable. To not be there when she needs help and support, or to hold her when she can't sleep because she needs you to tell her a bedtime story; there are no words to describe that pain. That night, I can imagine the sorry my aunt suffered as she wondered what was going to happen to her beautiful and innocent child when she's gone. I believe the more we are dependent on and emotionally attached to someone, the harder our farewell and the more difficult is to adapt to a new situation.

I knew she was suffering from cancer. I knew she was experiencing excruciating pain, even so, I couldn't let her go. Still, after 30-years, her memory scratches my heart and brings tears to my eyes. I was studying for my final year of school while she was in last days of her life. I recall her last look, how she nodded her head, signifying her despair and exhaustion from fighting cancer for so long. Tears ran down my cheeks and I fell asleep praying, trying to swallow my grief.

I saw her pale face in my dreams that night. She was wearing a long white dress and she gently patted my head. "Let me go," she said. "I am in pain, and you're keeping me here. Let me go." When I woke up, I felt calm. My beautiful aunty knew she was going to leave this mortal world and transcend to another realm. Despite wanting to be with her daughter, me, and the rest of the family, this was exactly what her spirit wanted. I didn't have any right to keep her here in pain. The day after my dream, I went shopping and bought myself a green scarf. Since then, it has become my ritual. Whenever I lose something, or have a big turning point in my life, I buy a colorful scarf.

In August 2020, I started my YouTube channel and later my podcast called "Transition by Pantea Kalhor".[5] I interviewed experts on fertility, loss, and struggle. It became so popular that my channel grew into a bigger platform where I met and interviewed amazing people who shared their own stories. One of my interviewees, Fiona Barr, a hypnotherapist, suggested I create a PTSD self-healing podcast. Before long, I did just that. I connected with amazing people who have gone on that same journey. I learned how they moved forward with their lives.

One Million Children Worldwide Have Lost a Parent to Covid, Study Finds."

This devastating news on Forbes[6] reminded me of my aunt and her farewell to her daughter. It motivated me to talk about grief in a different way, to look at it from another angle. I interviewed three women and one man who have gone down this difficult path and have included their stories in this book.

Coping with the sudden loss of a parent is a vast subject and could fill an entire book on its own. But I wanted to make sure there was room to include practical advice on how to use the different modalities to adapt to your new circumstances.

During a global pandemic, it's only natural that a lot of hidden post-traumatic stress symptoms arise. To lose loved ones and only be able to grieve in silence, not in person, is horrific. To be denied giving them the honour they deserve by holding a memorial service is breaking hearts around the globe. But for the sake of our kids, and all the survivors whose lives depend on us, all we can do is adjust to the new normal. To hold on to hope and create a better future by moving on.

# Erin Chandler Intuitive Guide and Psychic Medium

Meeting Erin Chandler was one of my fortunate coincidences; a beautiful, spiritual soul with a warm and clean vibration who has experienced the loss of her infant and overcame her battle through intuitive guidance. There is time for grief, a time for surrender, and a time for recovery.

We can't recover from loss completely because our memories remind us of all the sweet moments we have spent with our lost ones. It can keep us from moving forward, but we need to move past all those dark moments of grief, negative emotions, blame, and anger. We need to be alive and move on in our life to accomplish our mission until we join them in eternity.

Erin Chandler teaches others how to tap into their intuitive guidance and use their intuitive compass. She also educates others on how to connect with their loved ones on the other side and grieve with them instead of for them.

Listening to Erin's story aroused my emotions, touched my heart, and encouraged me to have her back for my PTSD summit. I asked her to share her story with you following her interview at the summit.[7]

**Erin Chandler's Story, Healing Grief and Trauma Through Intuitive Guidance and Healers:**

My journey started with the sudden death of my youngest daughter, Ava, back in 2010. That experience—my greatest loss—turned into my greatest purpose, the greatest of gifts, and the greatest healing.

We all know grief is a long journey, and it takes a lot of time to recover, if at all. In fact, I spent seven years not being able to grieve or express my sorrow and feelings. I saw different therapists, which were not always beneficial. I lost a lot of relationships and became unable to work. My health declined until I could barely get out of bed. I couldn't parent my children and my intimate relationships all fell apart. Being penniless led to the loss of my house and I got to the point where it felt like nobody could help me. I had no safe place to grieve. Nobody could figure out what was wrong with my health. It was like there were no answers for anything I was feeling, and eventually, I just couldn't do it anymore.

A person can only handle so much suffering and so much loss without an outlet or a safe place before it really becomes soul-crushing and hopeless. That's where I was. Grieving and utterly hopeless.

Early one morning, I went out into the middle of the forest by myself and spent time alone. It was time to plan how I would end my life. I felt I was of no benefit to anyone, and I couldn't function because the internal pain was so intense. It was so fierce that it manifested externally. I stopped walking and looked up at the sky.

"God, I give up," I said. I surrendered, and I felt better for it. A few days later, I got a call from an extended family member. Unbeknown to me and the family, she was a covert medium.

"Your daughter has been coming to me crying," she said. "She's saying that you gave up." Those were the exact words I had spoken aloud to God in the forest. No one knew that except me and God. No one in my family had any idea what was going on. As soon as she said those words, an enormous shift began. I was suddenly aware that my daughter was not gone. I believe we don't die, because if we do, there was no way she would have known what I'd said in the forest a short time earlier.

My desire to live sparked again. I knew Ava wasn't gone, that she would help me, that I wasn't forgotten, that I wasn't alone.

This conversation resulted in an immediate decision. I would not end my life. I had an immediate paradigm shift. Everything I believed to be true mustn't be true after all. That's when my healing journey began, and my daughter has helped me tremendously throughout the process. It's the reason I can channel and help so many struggling on the grief journey.

I began learning how to connect with her, not just to hear, feel, and see her, but to get a response that I understood, to have a fluid conversation with her. Ava spoke great truth that led to my healing. She led me to places and people I needed help from. She still brings me people to work with who have lost their loved ones. Sometimes Ava connects me with people in the strangest of places, like the grocery store. I believe our deceased loved ones want to speak to us. They will use a vessel or a person they can deliver a message through.

It has been a wild, humbling, and deeply healing journey. The two things that I've discovered on this path are that we suffer in grief because we feel our loved ones are gone, which leads to hopelessness. Yet the opposite is true. With so much evidence given through Ava and many other spirits, I now know that indeed they are not gone.

Our loved ones are literally just a thought away, closer to us than in life, and they want us to connect with them so that they may aid in the healing process. That evidence provides hope, which gives us the strength to keep living, to keep going.

I have done different modalities of therapy, like talk therapy, psychotherapy, and EMDR (Eye Movement Desensitization and Reprocessing). A psychotherapy treatment used to relieve the distress associated with trauma.

There are traditional modes of therapy that can help us move through trauma and grief. Some of those therapists I saw created even bigger barriers to healing than I came to them with. But once I found the right psychologist, several of these therapies were very effective.

I think the purpose of any method of therapy or healing modality should be to provide a safe space for us to express our experiences openly. Then guide us through and out the other side of it, allowing us to find purpose out of the pain. When I combined traditional psychology with spirituality and the ability to grieve with my daughter, instead of for her, it changed everything.

Absolutely nothing compares to having a full-on conversation with the person you think is gone from your life forever. There is nothing like having every conversation you never got to have, but wish you had. There is nothing like the feeling of pure love that one feels when they are connecting with their loved one in spirit.

In truth, I would never be able to help people in such a deep and profoundly healing way without mediumship and my spiritual faith. I would also never have found this much peace, this much love, truth, and healing, if it were not for my daughter teaching me how to connect with her and others' loved ones.

I believe everyone can connect. It's not a gift just for the few, but a gift for everybody. Everyone has a built-in intuitive compass and guidance system that is always available to them. With it comes the capability to hear, see, and/or feel their deceased loved ones with them all the time. They simply need to learn how to do this in a logical way.

The greatest healing happens when you realize you are indefinitely connected to them. Truly, this journey has been magical. Yes, it has been dark and painful and filled with great loss, but it has also been the most expansive, loving, and enlightening experience. The healing I have experienced within my spirit has alleviated more than just the weight of grief, depression, and dark pain associate with Ava's death. It has also changed the way many people view death and how they process grief.

### Erin's Recovery Solutions

Tapping into your soul is a requirement for any type of healing, whether it's trauma, PTSD, or grief. All modalities of healing are forms of self-care, ways of rebuilding trust in self. Then it expands into the external world and people again. The ultimate self care for healing is establishing a connection with yourself again. Through connecting with your loved ones in spirit, you build a new and stronger foundation of self and with the world.

When you learn how to have a conversation with the person you are grieving for, the one that has transitioned out of their body, it allows you to say everything you did not get to say. It allows you to heal all the wounds from the problems you didn't get to solve when they were alive. It is a profound type of healing when you get to grieve with your loved one instead of grieving for them.

When we think about mediumship or intuitive guidance, we often think of airy fairy, crystal balls, or the movie 'Ghost'. We have been conditioned to believe that mediums, psychics, and energy healers are not real, that they're a hoax or untrue. Yet the facts over the course of thousands of years and the recounts of millions of people's experiences prove otherwise. There is evidence that it is indeed real and very true. This becomes so obvious when I give others mediumship readings and intuitive guidance in their healing process.

Mediumship is about the living, not the deceased person they are coming to hear from. Our loved ones in spirit always want to talk about all the experiences that you have had. Like your current relationships, anything and anyone that hurt you, any wounds you are still carrying, both from childhood and throughout your life. It heals all wounds, not just one hurt, one relationship, or one loss. Our loved ones come to love and help heal everything within us.

There are many methodologies for healing that appeal to every taste, personality, and experience. I always encourage my clients to incorporate multiple types of therapy and self-care, whether it's art therapy, physical therapy, writing, or talk therapy. I believe we can and should mix and match, using the ones that suit each individual best. Anything that eases suffering helps us process and lighten our emotions or is in any way healing.

When we combine different healing modalities with the learned skill of tapping into our loved one's messages and universal guidance, the healing and transformation occurs in a much more rapid and profound way than just the traditional therapy methods.

The universe and our loved ones in spirit see every little horror and injustice that you have been through, whether we share it with another person or not. They want to lift you up and walk through the pain with you. They want to show you that you are not alone at all. That they are cheering you on, every single step of the way.

My daughter Ava and learning how to tap into the spirit realm have been profoundly healing for me. No traditional paths of therapy or psychology would ever have gotten me to where I am today. Connecting with my daughter and tapping into universal guidance is the reason I get up every day with more joy and passion than ever before. It's the reason I have been able to help so many others do the same. It's truly an honour to connect deeply with spirit and those who are on the life-changing journey of grief and loss.

# Nancy Nance, Recovery Coach

Nancy Nance is a survivor of loss and grief. Her story is about her daughter Emily, who was killed in a boating accident. What should a mother do after this misfortune? Nancy could have sought after something to numb her pain; something that could make her forget the reality, but after some time had passed, she found strength in her relationship with her son, who was also badly injured in that accident.

After a few years of seeking peace and trying different healing modalities to mend her broken heart and cope with her new situation, she finally found joy through her loss.

**Nancy Nance's Story, Finding Joy After Loss**

The day I experienced joy again was not a day I marked on my calendar. There was no formula that said in 322-days, and you'll be filled with happiness. My journey through grief was uncovering and understanding my feelings because I had shut down, stopped feeling.

I didn't know how to articulate my feelings. There were a lot of blue words I used to describe my feelings, the four-letter ones that start with b and f. But I kept telling everybody I was fine, that I was really good.

I was already using a library of coping mechanisms to heal my life before my daughter Emily passed in 2011. I went through the trauma of a 25-year abusive marriage and the drama of being in a chaotic, addictive, and co-dependent life. When I wrote my trauma ladder—the list of all the traumas that I've been through—I realized my life was not normal. Why would anybody sign up for this kind of existence?

After the accident, I was extremely angry. The hatred that was seething through my soul was so dark I believed death would feel better than life. I hated the driver of the boat who killed Emily. I couldn't go a day without being weighed down with depression and my anxiety was out control. As my marriage crumbled, I filled journal after journal with my thoughts. I was the only one willing to heal.

Then my granddaughter passed away within months of my divorce, and incredible sadness weighed upon me. I felt like life was supposed to be terrible, and terrible it was.

I knew I needed to heal. The only thing that made me feel better was yoga. So, I became a certified yoga teacher. I became bendy. I twisted and turned my body and continued to pose until I became better. I was okay, yet I still needed a lot more healing. Happiness seemed possible after I continued the healing process and practiced Reiki Self Healing.

I healed through layer after layer of hidden pent-up traumas. I learned about the incredible power of emotions and eventually I felt there was something better for me than the overwhelming hatred I had for life. That deep resentment was palpable. I hated waking up in the morning. But I continued to pursue healing.

I worked through my addiction to retail therapy that racked up my credit cards to distract myself from my feelings. I'd always wake up with that same dreadful feeling of being alive and knew I had to change. I promised my daughter that I would find a way to live again, and I didn't give up.

I found processes that worked and learned to understand the power of healing my deep trauma, and I embraced each area of pain. It didn't just suddenly turn me into a happy and optimistic person. I had to learn to work through each memory and heal the pain. To learn how to love life.

### Nancy's Recovery Solutions

Ask me about essential oils and you'll see her smile. I love how the power of nature can help heal the pain that life sometimes brings. I love the incredible power of smell. The healing power of oils is truly tremendous and the more I learn, the more I love to share. That's what makes me happy. It's a truly wonderful process. Add essential oils to meditation and you can transcend into an amazing place of peace.

Healing is possible for everyone. We just need to find someone that can help us navigate the path. When you struggle with any form of addiction, and everybody has struggled with some form of addiction in their life, you need to find understanding. Ask yourself what is missing in your life. When you experience trauma, digging deep into the subconscious pain will bring a deep healing to your soul. We all at some stage in our lives, strive to find pleasure in our life, whether that's from a bag of Twizzlers or something a little stronger, like a line of cocaine. But it won't numb the pain.

## Nancy's Final Words

*Quitters never win, and winners never quit.*

Most people have experienced some form of PTSD in their lives. It is the past trauma, stress, and drama that leads us to the amazing path to recovery. I have lived through the grief of losing precious love to find every lasting joy. I have struggled through the healing of abuse to understand the value of love.

I have created a process to help transform the pain, and I'd feel blessed, grateful, and excited if you'd let me help you recover from your loss.

# Richard Morden , Certified EFT Practitioner and Emotional Success Coach

Imagine you were just watched your wife die, but you needed to be a strong shelter for your kids who were grieving over the loss of their mom. There is no time to give up, there is no time to hide. As someone who'd already been down that road and experienced the loss of his parents and his siblings, Richard knew once again he had to show up for the rest of his family.

He also knew that he needed to work on all broken pieces of himself so he could be a good father. It was the only way he could protect his children and help them move on with their lives again.

Trauma isn't always obvious. PTSD can happen over a long period of time. It can compound subtly, such as from an abusive relationship, or from a sudden life-changing event. Richard had not just experienced sudden loss; he'd also lived through watching a loved one on their slow journey towards death. He sat by his mother's bedside for nine months after watching her suffer for 12-years. His wife also died of a brain aneurysm.

"We spend too much time fixing, and not enough time creating," Richard tells his clients. "We can create our lives with intention, and purpose, and release the resistance such as traumatic events. The key is creating, it keeps us inspired to always do more."

Richard Morden is also co-author of this book and has written a separate chapter to dig into EFT—Emotional Freedom Technique or the Tapping Method. This is his story.

**Richard Morden's story, How to Cope with the Loss of Your Family Member**

I witnessed my mother's journey with cancer from age 9 to 21 in 1978, with her final 9-months confined to a hospital bed. She was in the hospital several times throughout those years with chemotherapy. It wasn't until the last two years of her life that we knew she would not recover. I would go to work, then sit with her in the evenings to talk. However, talking wasn't an option in the final weeks of her life because the medications affected her mind.

I was completely unaware of how much of my life I had shut off. I had limited my expectations of anything better happening to me. I was already numb as a child from my father who traumatized all of us with his abusive behavior and violent rage. I was the youngest of six and had no way to help as I watched my sibling's self-destruct.

The two oldest became alcoholics and my oldest brother committed suicide. He had called me the day before and I had not returned the call. Whether this was the final straw, I will never know. When a mutual friend called me to say something had happened to him, I called the police. Their answer was a request to come in and identify his body.

It was a traumatic circumstance, yet I didn't understand it. I had no emotional response to it all at that time. That was 1988.

In 2013, my wife was a nurse and travelling with two coworkers to a conference when she went unconscious in the car. Being nurses, they knew what to do and immediately worked on her. They called an ambulance, which transported her to hospital. After receiving the phone call about her situation, I gathered up my children and her parents, and we rushed to the hospital in London, Ontario. We arrived around 11:00 p.m. and were ushered straight into her room.

It was a shock to see her on a ventilator lying so still. We met with the doctor an hour later and he told us they had performed two brain scans and determined that she was 90% brain dead. There was no hope of recovery, and I knew in that second, I was going to have to take her off life support.

I turned to my kids, and both sets of parents.

"We need to let her go," I said. I didn't want to let her go, but the decision to set her free wasn't difficult after witnessing my mother's long battle. I see it now as a blessing in disguise as the brain aneurysm happened quickly, so she didn't have to endure pain.

Our children did not see her suffer, so that was a good thing. However, this happened just before my daughter's graduation from high school. These things happen in life, but we were lucky to have a good family unit with my in-laws, so there was support among us and with my extended family. I was in grief, but I didn't recognize the accumulation of the trauma I had. No one else knew I had suffered from depression for years. I functioned fine in the working world.

But as I watched my siblings self-destruct, I could see that I was different. Their journey was not my journey. They did drugs and alcohol, and somehow, I had the sense I needed to stay true to my body.

So, I went to the gym where I felt I had some control and expectation of hope for my life. Lifting weights and focusing on simple movements—as I call it, 'Push & Pull'—the gym took a lot of rage out of me. I was also working on a farm, so I pushed myself to exhaustion. My system was so full of energy I was able to work twelve-hour days and then a two-hour workout at the gym.

I knew I needed to focus on self-care so I could be present for my children. Then in October, I found EFT (Emotional Freedom Technique) and went on a three-day course. I had two massive traumas released from my body that weekend, one from my father and the other from my brother's suicide. It was like a volcano. I was sweating and almost vomited. I had so much energy, like someone pulling hot lava out of your body.

"This is huge for me," I said. "There's got to be more." So, I took the course again in the spring with Nancy Forrester, who is a Master EFT trainer and founder of Conscious EFT. I signed up for her 10-month course, 'Harness your Power'. Nancy is also a psychotherapist, now retired. In the course, we really focused on self-care and doing our own work. I fell in love with the process because there were a lot of unresolved traumas that needed to be processed. It was such a blessing to work with colleagues.

It's an ongoing process, but the pieces fell into place and allowed me to be present for my children. That's why I am so grateful. I allowed myself to be present and my children moved on very well in their life. I take credit for the part I played, but I was also lucky enough to have a supportive family that cared for them and kept in contact on a continual basis.

Now, my son has become a nurse and after university, my daughter worked for a while, and then wanted to travel. I was all for it but wanted to make sure she was going for the right reasons.

"Are you running away?" I asked.

"No," she said.

"Would you go if your mom was still alive?"

"No."

"Would you go if your grandma was alive?"

"No. But they've both passed away now."

I understood that and told her I'd see her later and wished her a good life.

If her mother or grandmother were alive, she would have stayed local and tried to live her life to please them. So many people do this thinking it's the right thing to do and then have very unhappy lives and don't know why. It's because they never went after things that were significant to them.

In February 2014, I wrote on paper what I wanted my new relationship to look like. In 2016, I met my dream girl, and we have been together since then. She is a medium as well. So, we have a great relationship. She talks to spirits and to me. I don't know who she is talking to sometimes, but there is always lots of chatter going on in the house. I was very clear on how I wanted my new relationship to feel, so I wrote it all down. That's how I am living today. We learn to create our lives by the way we think and the intentions and emotions we have towards your goals.

**Richard's Recovery Solutions**

We were required to do our own personal peace procedure when we took the EFT course. That was a big part of uncovering the layers of trauma as well. I guess for me, it's the resilience we gain on the journey. I've always been a guy who just woke up and went to work at my job, so it was just work for me. My desire was to be present for myself and my children, so that was my focus. I just used different modalities along the way and all of it is like pearls on a chain. One person gets you over the hump and it feels like the miracle, but the most significant part of the healing journey is the relationships you create with others. Every person, every experience, adds to your journey until you can thrive. I have done thousands of hours of tapping on myself and with clients.

I've been dedicated to my own healing work because I knew I couldn't be there for my clients if I had something that was being triggered in me. It's fun because when you embrace your journey and look at where you were at the beginning and where you are now, you can see how much progress you've made. Give yourself praise for that. You are worthwhile. Accept it when someone else says nice things about you.

We're all on a journey. We just have to plug into it so we can thrive.

# CHAPTER 2: Healing Perinatal Trauma

The pain that stabbed my belly felt like I'd been pierced with a bowie knife. Then the blood loss started. Yet again, another cycle had failed. I've been through this twice before.

Miscarriage hurts. It's an amalgamation of grief from the loss, feeling imperfect like you're faulty somehow, desperate, or unworthy.

When you first hear that fast rhythm of a heartbeat, you get excited about becoming a mother. But then the heart stops beating, and you feel dead inside your womb. All the sweet dreams of hugging your baby in your arms are replaced with the nightmare of pain and blood loss.

Every time I lost a baby, the agony hit like something was separating inside not just from my body, but from my soul. After two years of struggling with recurrent miscarriages, I knew I had to change something in me if I was to break the cycle.

In the I.T. world we have something called an infinite loop. There is no breaking condition defined. As humans we can end up repeating the same pattern repeatedly unless we find an exception.

In my case, I gave up medication and tried holistic remedies and acupuncture. I learned that even if we are stuck in an unpleasant cycle of failure, we need to stop the process and find an alternative approach to healing. If you are interested in following my healing story on how I stopped the vicious cycle of miscarriage and gave birth to my daughter, you can read my third book: *Naturally Conceived: How to Get Pregnant, Explain Unexplained Infertility and Prevent Miscarriages by Unleashing Your Reproductive Power Even Over 40!* [8].

# Linda Hayes Cooper Early Parenting Therapist, Clinical Psychologist, Hypnotherapist, and NLP Practitioner

I have interviewed Linda Hayes Cooper four times in different shows. Such a lovely and supportive lady with a noble mission. She is the advocate for early parental loss and miscarriages; she teaches how to shift parents' mindset so that they can prepare for future pregnancies using methods that create calmness and safety. Linda has also written a separate chapter in this book, analyzing her case study.

**Linda Hayes Cooper's Story, Healing Prenatal Trauma**

As a clinical psychologist with a focus on perinatal care, I met many new and expectant parents with various mood disorder symptoms. Initially, my previous work was in midwifery. I worked in a large teaching hospital, so I was familiar with what traumatized women experienced. It was always very medicalised and at times it was hard to practice the natural way I wanted to practice.

I used to see a lot of women going through trauma after the birth. But it wasn't until I was doing private home visits later that I realized there are a lot of women still talking about their births. Some said they were having dreams, nightmares, even flashbacks of the midwife's or obstetrician's voice that they would never forget.

It was clear these women were still feeling traumatized, even suffering from PTSD. I had women coming in before and after the birth, and I was surprised at how they could focus so deeply on the event. They could feel and experience it all over again. It wasn't about the event; it was really about their emotional perception of what happened. That's when I started working with both moms and dads to help them manage their grief and loss after things didn't go quite to plan.

It was talk therapy that held the most value for them. I helped them face their emotions and be present in their body and slowly experience their feelings. So many relive the event over and over. Yet when people asked them how they were, they didn't get the chance to experience those real emotions or talk about how they felt. Many couldn't be honest with how they were feeling now.

Rather than masking their feelings, these women needed to take some time to go through the process of talking, experiencing the emotion, and acknowledging their pain. Although this was difficult, it was extremely valuable. Eventually, they acknowledged they had the power and strength within them to be present to make the changes necessary simply by moving slowly and looking after themselves with compassion.

## Linda's Recovery Solutions

I haven't suffered from PTSD, although my last marriage was quite traumatic for me. After 12-months of silence from him, he left suddenly and went straight into another relationship. I pieced everything together, realizing that he had been building another relationship to step into for a long time.

It seemed that distancing himself from me made it easier for him to make the sudden break. I was in complete shock. I spoke with a psychiatrist friend and asked where health professionals go to get help when they felt like just driving into a pole because life wasn't worth living.

"Well, you're in shock," he said, "and it's New Year's Eve soon. I think you need to go somewhere safe." So, I admitted myself into a unit which, fortunately, had a nice, quiet room. I spent a lot of time doing crafts, coloring, writing, and meditating. All of which I absolutely loved. They were very therapeutic for me, especially meditation. It was a practice I had used previously with clients and myself, and it really centered me.

I did a lot of talk therapy, and I joined their yoga group as well as other activities. I integrated different elements or parts of my brain, along with eating healthily, and drinking plenty of water. They all provided an element of self-compassion.

Such a personal trauma took some time to get over. Working through this process was significant when it came to gaining the healing I needed. It then became something I could share with my clients occasionally to resonate with them when traumatized by their experiences. Especially when they were experiencing suicidal ideation. I could tell them of the many places they could go to get help. We don't have to be alone; we just need to reach out.

I still use all those techniques; however, in addition, I've been using a more spiritual, preventative approach. I hope to be practicing as one of the new pioneers in Prenatal Bonding (BA), which was put together by Janoe Raffai back in the late '80s or early '90s. Along with his student Dr. Gerhard Schroth—a psychiatrist in Germany—they use a preventative approach with women and partners in their pregnancy, in which they tap mothers into their own past grievances, traumas, and trans-generational patterns. They use Holding Space Hypnotherapy, regression work, and help them create a deeper connection with their babies.

The babies "talk" to their mothers. They communicate jointly. A combined international study found that out of 8,000 women using this practice, less than 1% had medical interventions with forceps or caesarean sections and suffered postpartum depression. Labour and birthing were easier and shorter. They had happy, bright, intelligent babies that were easygoing, well bonded, and well-connected with their families. [9]

# CHAPTER 3: How to Recover from a Consecutive Series of Trauma

Sometimes we fall victim to a series of traumas, one right after another. That might be rooted in abandonment or from being traumatized or bullied in childhood. It could be from getting stuck in an abusive relationship or from losing your loved ones.

You might be exhausted from being traumatized, but you don't want to give up. You just want to end the cycle of chronological traumas and feel happy and liberated. But you don't know how to start.

The big turning point in my life was when I was attacked and badly injured by the car thief, then had my fertility struggle and recurrent miscarriages. Migrating to two different countries, trying to cope with all the stress involved with relocating, along with some relationship traumas (until I found the love of my life), it all compounded.

All I could do was learn how to adapt and rise again. With every struggle, I grew more experienced, became more educated, and more energized. I've always loved living and thriving. I know that if I am breathing, if I can see the sky above, another day will come, and I will see another horizon, I will live through another season. If you are interested in reading my life story, you can find it in amazon: "Rules of Change for the Better: Real stories and your guide to tune-up your mood and transform your life to reach your biggest dreams." [10]

# Dr. Lizette Bataille Medical Director and Best-Selling Author

I interviewed Liz in my Authors Promotion Show to talk about her book: *Life Launch: Surviving the Storms of Physical and Sexual Abuse*[11].

Dr. Liz knows what it's like to experience trauma, abuse, and grief. Her experiences with loss from sexual abuse, addiction, and suicidal ideation taught her that hope will get you back to a life that you love again.

Throughout her work with professionals and a 12-step program, she survived her traumas and found the strength to move forward with hope. Her purpose drives her desire to help others find peace and joy in their life after surviving trauma. At the ARISE! Mind, Body, Spirit Healing Institute, Dr. Liz provides holistic healing strategies, education, and practices to thrive beyond trauma, abuse, addiction, or suicidal ideation. Her healing exercises awaken the mind, body, and spirit to a new joy of life. With 30-years in the medical field, Dr. Liz is well educated in the workings of the human body and the healing practices that get things back on track. She's an international best-selling author with her first nonfiction book, *Life Launch - Surviving the Storms of Physical and Sexual Abuse, Book One.*

## Healing after Her Husband's Suicide

The most traumatic experience occurred when I was forty-two years old. I had been married for three and a half years. It had been five and a half years since we met and started dating, and we had a child that was two years and 10 months old.

It was Friday night and my husband, 27, and I, 15-years his senior, were going to head to Disney World with our son, who was about to turn three. I drove home from the town up north where I worked and stopped to pick up our son. The next stop was to pick up my husband. I'd already done the packing for our weekend away, so I was excited and ready to go.

I went into the house to get him and felt what I understood later to be the very definition of dead silence. It was 16-years ago now, but I can still see it all as if it only happened yesterday. The light was on in the garage, so I yelled in that direction.

"Hey, are you ready? What are you doing?" As I walked towards the garage, I kept asking questions.

"Are you getting the clothes down from the attic?"

I rounded the corner into the garage, and there he was, hanging from the rafters. I rushed to him. I had to save him. There was no one else around to help me. He was still warm, and as I struggled to get him down, I remember thinking he was going to get the air knocked into him when he dropped.

However, none of that happened. I must have screamed because my neighbor arrived and together, we tried to revive him by giving him CPR. On most Friday nights in Florida, everybody goes outside to get ready for the evening, so it wasn't long before the other neighbors came. But it was too late. He was gone.

That was the beginning of a whole new life for me. Being 42-years old with a toddler made me feel like my life was over. It was the worst time in the world for me. The worst time in my life.

When I spoke to my spiritual advisor, which was part of my healing process, he said that I was going through a dark time of transition. My life as I knew it was over, and I didn't have any clue what my new life was going to be like. All I could see waiting ahead for me was darkness, sadness, and gloom.

I've talked to a lot of people about suicide. It's one thing to have a loved one do that when you're not there to find them. But it's goes to a whole other level if you are the one who actually finds them. I think that's where the post-traumatic stress came from.

Unfortunately, I have had many other types of traumas in my life, too. I talked about everything with my spiritual advisor, especially how I going to get a new life when my old life has gone. It was a horrible place to be in - that dark in-between place.

The acknowledgement from him that he knew and understood where I was at, was so important. He got the fact that I knew my old life was gone and I couldn't see my new life yet. So, over the next 10 years, I did all the things I'd done previously that had worked. I used all the knowledge I'd gleaned while going through mental addiction and through the grieving process after the deaths of my brother and dad.

I had been using chiropractic and massage therapy to help, but I kept researching and found a few therapies worth trying. Some of which helped me a lot. One was acupuncture, another was color therapy, and they both worked. Color therapy is important. I continue with many of these practices today.

I had never really tried aromatherapy before, but it worked. I also tried equine therapy. I know a lot of veterans use therapy riding for their PTSD. A care provider who was administering the equine therapy told me it was extremely helpful. I was delighted when it worked for me as well. And finally, ten years after my husband's death, the last thing I tried—and it's not like it was more important than the others, but it just got me over the hump—was Feng Shui.

Another part of my message to you is not to scoff at something that somebody else is suggesting to you. I would never have thought that taking a mirror out of my bedroom would have completely lifted 10-years of grief off my shoulders, but it did. Mirror reflects back to you all the emotions it absorbs.

I was crying during the day. At night, when I was sleeping right across the bed from my mirror, that sadness was coming back on me. I thought, well, heck, I'm going to try that, and I took that mirror out of the bedroom. The next morning, I felt like I began to live my life again. Once again, I loved my life. I am not saying that Feng Shui is more powerful than anything else I tried, but it is powerful.

My ability to get on the other side of my grief was due to the cumulative effect of all 50 different therapies that I'd implemented since my teen years.

I remember reading that people who commit suicide try a hundred different things first. Apparently, there's a list of these things. It's not like they literally go down this list. But I understand that they're just trying to find something that makes them feel better. Eventually, many take the one act that ends their life. It is not a choice, and it is not a decision.

I feel like that's what I did on my healing journey. I kept trying to find the thing that helped me feel better. Suicidal ideation is a big part of my story, too, and that's probably why I ended up finding my late husband.

I tried 50 different healing strategies and listed them in my Healing Resources booklet, which you can find my website. For me, every single thing, I put into practice culminated in getting on the other side of the grief, to truly wanting to LIVE my life again. You can do it too. That is the most important message I want to share with you. If you're feeling hopeless or suffering from a mental illness, never give up. Try everything until you find what works for you. I did, and that is what I attribute my healing to.

# CHAPTER 4: Combat PTSD, Military Sexual Trauma (MST)

Looking at soldiers who have deployed to a battlefield may remind you of numerous Hollywood movies. You may admire them for their bravery and see them as people who earn medals and defeat the enemy. But what you may never imagine is how much damage war can cause them. How difficult it is for them to see their buddy's head or limbs explode in front of them. In war, they experience the toughest experiences of loss and death that a human can ever withstand.

Eight years of my childhood was lived in fear. Fear that a bomb would drop on us. I remember trying to survive, escaping from one city to another trying to stay safe. My mind can still recall the sound of a raid alert broadcasting over the radio. We knew that night, the death lot would fall upon a family.

In order to survive, we had to shelter in the basement. We had to wait and see what our destiny held. Whether we'd survive another night. As the bombs fell, we tried to handle the stress by using our sense of humor. It kept our hopes and dreams alive and helped us visualize a bright future.

War is bitter and the impact of the damage remains with so many for years. All the children affected by the war will always remember the tragedy. Their bodies store that pain at the cellular level. Pregnant women transfer the fear of survival to their fetus, and those babies who are born in war will have a trace of fear, famine, death, and loss in their memories unless they can reframe their life and redefine their existence.

I don't like any movies that have war-scenes, bombing, or a battlefield in them. It still triggers me. I always ask myself why we, as adults, still can't live a life in peace? Why do people still live in the countries where there is still war? I know the answer. Do you? Let's be hopeful that one day we all live in harmony, peace, and unity and no vicious power rules the world.

We, as a whole, like body organs, are connected to each other. When I see the happiness of a family, the cheerful giggling of little kids, a white wedding dress and romantic smiles exchanging between the happy couple, an ultrasound of a fetus inside the womb, the excitement of a child playing on a playground, I am thrilled because I know this joy is going to be added to the happiness of the entire world.

In holistic medicine, healing starts from within when we feel happy and at peace inside. The headache is only a symptom, but the root-cause could be related to any part of the body. The wisdom of the world feels the pain of its organs, and by the time there is war, famine, exploitation, and manipulation, the world suffers injustice. I am hopeful one day we will all unite and live peacefully together by enjoying our differences.

I am going to gift this chapter to brave veterans who are fearlessly fighting for peace and defending their countries. I just want to tell them I can understand their pain as a sister who has spent her childhood in war, even if she has never fought on a battlefield.

I could empathize with Roseline Salazar, a retired Air Force Military Officer, now a PTSD coach. While I was interviewing her in my PTSD Self-Healing Show and PTSD summit, I knew the real meaning of war. Roseline is a wife and mother of two beautiful children. Her deployments as an officer included Afghanistan, Iraq, and Saudi Arabia in her enlisted days. Roseline has since been diagnosed with combat PTSD and is also a military sexual trauma (MST) survivor. She is a certified mental health coach now, helping others realize and learn that there is life after the military, and life after trauma.

# Roseline Salazar Workplace Bullying, and Combat PTSD

My military experience includes going on convoys, completing battlefield circulations, and making supply runs. We never knew what the day would bring. Our camp was attacked and once, two rocket mortars flew just 10 feet over my head. I still remember clear as day how we were ambushed during one of our supply runs. We got stuck in downtown Khost. The worst part was always when we lost people.

On top of the rocket attacks and the convoy ambush, the hardest to bear was when our own men turned against me because my boss was bullying me.

He'd liked me, actually became obsessed with me. But since I didn't reciprocate those feelings, he used his rank and intimidation to make my life a living hell. He threatened everyone who talked to me until no one dared. I felt so alone, so isolated. He also mentally abused me by saying I was worthless, that no other sections would take me on because I was lazy. None of these were true.

When I didn't do what he wanted, the beatings started. Every day was difficult. While out on convoys, we never knew if we were going to survive another day or live long enough to make it home to our families.

During this time, I called my mom every day. She was my biggest supporter and guardian angel, who prayed for us to stay strong and healthy, and for our safe return home. Sadly, she passed away two years ago.

With everything going on, the isolation, the abuse, and not knowing if I was going to see another day, I became so overwhelmed; I attempted suicide. I downed the entire bottle of Ambien CR—the medication prescribed to help me sleep—hoping I could escape the hell and not wake up the next morning. I was desperate to make it all stop.

That night, we got attacked, and since I didn't report to my assigned bunker, my boss came to my bedroom with some co-workers, and they found me. They carried me outside and I had to wake up run to the MRAP vehicles (Mine-Resistant Ambush Protected vehicles) and drive. But that wasn't my lowest point. While watching the convoy leave our camp on the office camera, I witnessed and heard the ambush on the convoy. Our First Sergeant's head was hit by a rocket-propelled grenade and because everyone had believed my boss when he previously said I was weak and stupid, I was blamed for his death.

Thank God I had an awesome roommate who prayed with me. Although at first, I didn't want her to because I was mad at God.

"That's who you need to turn to right now, because we can't even trust our own people," she said. So, we prayed every day, followed by 30-minute meditation sessions. She also taught me breathing techniques, told me to pray before going on supply runs, and to look forward to seeing my family when I got back.

It wasn't easy at the time, but it worked. Praying, meditating, the breathing exercises, and having a picture of my family to go home to, is what got me through. I reminded myself continually that I had six months left and that I'd get through this. And that's what I did.

I launched a complaint about being bullied by the leadership. Turns out that the leadership was aware of my situation, but they hadn't protected me or rectified the situation. Then I was told it was my fault because I allowed it to happen.

After waiting three months for the outcome, I lost the case because I wasn't given a lawyer to represent my case. I felt defeated and lost all hope in our military and government system. I never received the justice I deserved. My boss won, he got away with all his wrongdoings, and was able to remain in active duty. I was medically retired after being diagnosed with PTSD. They said I wasn't mentally fit to serve anymore.

I continued therapy and other treatments. It took me 10-years before I could even start living life like I used to. My kids were my saving grace and motivation to move on. I kept reminding myself that their lives depended on me, that I need to set the example and raise them right. Through therapy, breathing exercises, and meditation, I found peace and justice for myself by accepting the past.

My primary outlet for my feelings was writing a book about my experiences using coping techniques. They're what helped me get to where I am today. My goal is to help those without a voice, both females and males, who were wronged—like myself—and encourage them that there is life after the military.

By being able to share my experiences legally, and remind myself how far I'd come, that I was safe now, I got through the toughest time in my life.

**Roseline Salazar - Solution**:

I still practice mindfulness and have learned to live in the present, not in the past, so I can focus on my future.

Roseline has added a separate chapter in this book and has talked more deeply about her journey and, especially, her solution modalities.

# CHAPTER 5: Abusive Relationships and Domestic Violence

Sometimes life strangles you in a bottleneck and doesn't let you move. The glitter of a romantic attraction steals your heart, and you believe in love. Then, while playing with those love cards, another game is revealed to you. You notice your dreamland was just a seductive mirage, a lie, a stifling vortex. You flounder and try to get out of the whirlwind, but it feels like you sink deeper and deeper every day.

You try hard to stay in that relationship by tolerating the disrespect, humiliation, accusation, manipulation, emotional and physical abuse, because you believe your love is strong. But that 'one day' you'd been promising yourself, that future where everything was going to be fine, it never arrives. The cycle of abuse repeats and it gets worse. Much worse.

I was watching a series on Netflix called *Maid,* which depicts the life of a young mother with a dysfunctional family, an alcoholic partner, and a beautiful 3-year-old daughter. The young mother worked as a maid, cleaning houses at minimum wage in order to make ends meet and be able to take the custody of her daughter.

It took her a few attempts to get out of the relationship with her abusive partner. She had to get governmental support and live in a shelter that accommodated domestic violence survivors. The woman who managed the shelter told her that sometimes it takes up to 7-attempts before most women can finally set themselves free and get out that cycle of abuse. In some cases, the abuser is cunning enough not to leave any sign of physical injury, making it difficult to prove the abuse. However, sometimes emotional insult is more damaging than receiving a physical thrashing.

When you suffer from PTSD, having kids complicates the situation. You may need to go through the courts to get child custody, and then all the responsibility of raising your kids is on you. The finances, managing their tantrums, trying to be the mom and the dad is tough. Especially while you're still on the journey to recovery.

This subject on relationship trauma and domestic violence can fill the entire book. But its main purpose is to give you examples of life events the trauma experts have experienced, and their processes used to find healing. They now help others to shift their mindset and step into the recovery process with more confidence. Finding support groups and getting the right guidance will also be of great help to you in your journey of recovery.

# Maricelly Ramos Life Coach

Maricelly Ramos is a domestic violence survivor. The first time I met her, I saw a confident woman with a strong voice and a powerful story. I admire her for how she's taken control of her life. She is a mother who had to stay in an abusive relationship for the sake of protecting her children. But it all got too much, and she realized enough is enough. She took the plunge and became a single mom who has raised her kids on her own.

After 15-years, she rallied the strength to write her book. She is now an author, certified life coach, and entrepreneur. Sometimes after we leave a relationship, we don't know where to start. Maricelly helps women reconnect with themselves after the cycle of abuse.

**Maricelly Ramos' Story - Surviving an Abusive Relationship**

I saw the effects of domestic violence as a child watching my mother being abused. So, I grew up thinking that was normal. But my personal story started when I was fifteen. I met this man who, at a time, was still married with a child. For some reason, he kind of just came into my life and we started dating.

In some cultures, age difference doesn't really matter, so I was okay with it. At first, we had no problems. But it didn't take long before the control began. I wasn't allowed to spend time with my friends or make new ones. I couldn't wear certain clothes if he didn't approve of them.

A few months into the relationship, he started the physical abuse. He wouldn't just tap or push me. He punched, grabbed my neck, and pulled out my hair. This abusive behaviour lasted for many years. It's like I kind of got addicted to it. I was young and had no one to give me guidance, plus I thought it was normal. The relationship with my mother wasn't strong enough for me to tell her what he was doing, how he was abusing me.

By the time I turned eighteen, I moved out of my family's home and moved in with him. I thought because of that, he was going to change. He did, but not in the way I'd hoped. The abuse and terror escalated. It was just me and him, so he was free to drag me around the floor and treat me any way he wanted.

"If you fall asleep, and I catch you asleep, then it's going to be your last night," he said on numerous occasions. So, I found the courage to get a knife and hide it under my bed. I lived in fear, wondering if I was going to get any sleep that night, and if I would even wake up in the morning.

Being in an abusive relationship is like walking on ice, waiting, knowing that one day it was going to crack. *Am I going to make it through today? Is today going to be my last day on earth?* These are the questions I asked myself on a daily basis.

When you're being abused, it's normal to become suicidal. I didn't want to live anymore, not like that. Yes, I loved my children, but it got too much for my body and mind to cope with. It had to stop, and I was the only one who could make it happen.

So finally, I decided to become my own hero. I finally had the strength to call the police. I moved out and lived in a shelter, but I didn't heal. What I did instead was find someone else. He was even worse. It was the same pattern of physical and emotional abuse, the same controlling ways, the same power he exerted over me.

Not only did he hurt me, but he also started in on my daughter. When I found out he assaulted her sexually, it was like a big rock fell on top of me. I blamed myself and didn't handle things properly. So, my life fell apart. I turned to alcohol, then I moved out. Every day I kept thinking I was ready to heal, but I wasn't. I was stuck in a vicious cycle. Thinking suicidal thoughts, drowning my sorrows in more alcohol. I felt like I was going crazy. Then I couldn't help my children because I'd become so unhealthy. I was an empty cup.

Once again, I found the strength to move on. I finally met someone who I thought was a good person, and we got married. Soon after the wedding, he became emotionally abusive. He started his controlling behaviour. He took up drinking alcohol, but this time I wasn't going to allow it. I'd had enough.

That's when my reactive abuse began. Now, I wanted to put my hands on him. But one day I stopped and asked myself if I wanted to continue living this way. Did I want to live the rest of my years like this? The answer was no.

I started going to church. I started praying to God like I had never prayed before. "Please, God, can you hear me? Do you see me crying? Do you really want me to live like this? Is this how I'm going to live for the rest of my life?"

That's when he helped me find the strength. We separated soon after and I started getting therapy. I began praying regularly and apologized to my precious children. The consequences of my choices meant I had to build my relationship with them all over again. How was I going to get to know my children when I didn't even know myself? I had lost who I was, and I needed to learn to love myself.

Plus, I didn't know how to be a mom because I didn't have a mom who taught me how to love and be loved. I didn't know what a healthy relationship looked like, or how to love someone because I wasn't loved as a child. I had to learn step by step and it was frustrating because I couldn't fix it all in one day.

I found solace in writing. I wrote my memoir, and it brought back all trauma I'd been through. It was so difficult to write about. I filled the book with the emotions I'd experienced. Then when I lost a family member at the same time—someone who had always been like a brother to me—I found myself back in the grieving process again.

I kept writing, but it was difficult to talk about all those emotions. A lot of family members weren't happy about the book because it exposed what my mother had done to me growing up. So, I really didn't have any support. But one day after I published it, I got an email.

"I read your book and it has inspired me," it said. That made me feel like it was all worth the pain. I had learned so much and now I could help the voiceless and the hopeless on their journey. To tell them there is a light at the end of the tunnel, and if I did it, you can too.

**Maricelly's Solution**

The first thing I did was accept the things that happened to me. Once I'd done that, I identified my triggers. One thing that used to really bother me was having people stand behind my back. Even if I was just eating in my safe space, I always heard things behind me.

"Are they going to come and get me?" I thought. "Are they going to grab me from behind?" I didn't want to live that way, so I chose to change my thought patterns. I changed the internal dialogue.

"I'm in my safe place. Nothing is going to happen to me."

The more I told myself that, the more I believed it. Every time I felt anxious, like someone was going to grab me from behind, I'd talk to myself.

"You've got this. You are in your safe place."

I started writing a journal and in it are affirmation notes I speak over myself every morning.

"I am loved. I am worthy."

There are a lot of breathing techniques I do that help me. I listen to a lot of music, and I read a lot. I'm still writing too. I know I can't change my past, but I can build a new life for myself. So, now, I am finally able to look forward to my future.

# Dr. Lizette Bataille, Medical Director

I talked about Dr. Lizette Bataille in another chapter, but since her second story was more related to theme of this chapter, I added her story here.

**Dr. Lizette Bataille's story on abusive relationships**

My first experience with domestic violence was in my family home watching my parents' relationship. It was physically violent and verbally abusive, and so it was just normal, everyday life for me. They did not spare the rod, so to speak. They hit us. I guess they call it corporal punishment.

My mother would just backhand me if she didn't like what I said. She was often violet physically. I put my hands up to defend myself, or grab her wrists, and then she'd pull away and grab at my hair.

I remember when I was in my teens, and I felt guilty about pulling her hair back, but it was the only thing I could think of to make her let go. She didn't have any guilt about doing it. I wrote down that classic question: *How did I end up here?*

I swore to myself when I was 15-years old that I would never be like my parents. But 20-years later, when I was in my mid-30s, I still used them as negative role models. I ended up in a relationship just like that. I wasn't the perpetrator, which I thank God for. I didn't perpetrate the aggression, but I ended up with a violent man who did.

When I was 6-years sober, I found myself on the ground with my fiancé's hands around my neck. His knees were on my shoulders, pinning me down, and his fist was raised above my face, and this horrible feeling came over me.

"How did I get here? You should be well enough by now," I asked myself. It shows you the power of being a product of our environment; of what we learn.

'Children learn what they live'.

My first husband slapped me once, and I said, "Don't ever do that again." It was the second violent relationship I found myself in. After that, I never got involved in any relationship like that again. This is when my healing process started. This is where I started drawing the line.

I went onto the Internet to learn what constitutes 'Abuse' and 'Domestic Violence'. The first search result said that the abuser starts with name-calling. My parents were very good at that. I never thought that name-calling was verbal abuse.

So, from that day forward, that's where I drew the line. As soon as anybody called me a name, it didn't matter what the reason was; it was over. It's still a deal breaker for me today. I don't show people disrespect by name-calling, and I won't tolerate it being done to me. That one decision has helped me stay out of any type of unhealthy relationship.

### Dr. Lizette Bataille's Solution

Here's what I've learned in three parts:

First, if you're in an abusive relationship and need to get out, or you've already left and are now on the road to recovery, don't try to do it alone. Don't try to walk your journey without having somebody else to help you, whether it's a professional or a trusted friend.

Second, you must walk through the valleys in your journey. You can't go around them, or under them, and you definitely can't avoid them. Even through the dark times, even through the pain, keep walking. It doesn't matter whether you have a trusted friend on the journey, or if you are seeing a professional regularly, it's the working through it together that gives us hope.

Third, there is a quote in *The Big Book of AA* that I love so much.

***What at first, I thought was a flimsy read, was the loving and caring hand of God.***

Every time I think about it, it chokes me up. Because you never know where that help is coming from. I apologize for saying God if that's not what you believe. If you prefer, you could replace God with hope. It's been those three important keys that have helped me get through it all. Now, I have created a better life for myself.

# Jessica De Serre Boissonneault, Flight attendant, Best-selling Author

From a small town to a global inspiration; Jessica's story is inspiring. A few years ago, she left an abusive marriage and had to raise her daughter as a single mom. But it's what has helped her become the woman she is today.

Jessica has been a flight attendant for the past 11-years, certified NLP Practitioner, and three times international best-selling author. Her third book *I'm a Flight Attendant & That is my Superpower* launched on June 7th, 2021.

She is a woman empowerment advocate and has founded the "Women Empowerment Wednesday Show." She is also the founder of "Women in Power" the online virtual events which she will eventually host in person.

Jessica is also the founder of "Take Flight Academy", which will start officially in 2022, offering a 90-day coaching program, and much more. This program will teach the seven empowerment steps to live your best life.

**Jessica De Serre Boissonneault's story- Rising After an Abusive Relationship**

I was in an abusive marriage. I chose to be with that man, and I chose to get married and fall pregnant. I had my daughter and I say that my daughter saved my life because that's when that lioness inside of me woke up.

There was no way I was going to put my daughter in that situation. My mom did not raise me in that kind of environment. I was not exposed to violence or drugs, and I wouldn't allow my daughter to live that way.

I left when she was only 12-months old, and I knew it was going to be difficult. But I had to be strong for her. Turns out, it was the most traumatic time of my life.

Amongst the massive upheaval of becoming a young, single mom escaping domestic violence, I learned to heal myself. Then I realized I wanted to elevate other women. To teach them how to really live in their power, in their passion, and unbending positivity. Because life is so short. We don't know when our last day here will be.

Looking back, it all seems so clear now. My life happened exactly the way it needed to. That trauma led me to invest in myself; and from my full cup, I can now help you fill yours.

I always tell people my favorite quotes.

***Rock bottom became the solid foundation I built my life on. Unknown***

***I had to be broken, to be rebuilt, to be the woman that I am today. Jessica DSB***

One of the main things I want to encourage you with today is to understand the importance of investing in yourself. You cannot help others until you first help yourself. So, get the help you deserve. You are worth it.

On an airplane they always play the emergency videos first before take-off. They state you must 'Put your oxygen mask on FIRST, before you put it on your children." This is the same for life. Take care of you.

Rescue yourself first. The biggest investment you ever make should be in yourself. So, invest!

My entire life turned around when I started working with a coach and took several personal development courses with Landmark. That enabled me to surround myself with successful mentors.

Have you heard the expression "We're like onions" before? I started peeling some of my layers off and then realized my first trauma occurred the day I was conceived. My mom was only nineteen and she didn't want to have me. Luckily for me, she was against abortion. She felt trapped and obligated to see the pregnancy through. I experienced that in her belly, along with everything going on with my dad, who was using drugs.

From that moment on, my experience with life was toxic and unhealthy. As a result, and without realizing it at the time, my brain was being programmed.

"I'm not loved," and "I'm not important."

That trauma was carried with me through life, which affected my decision making. I ended up with the same type of men and they treated me poorly.

The biggest gift I gave myself was the choice I made to face the trauma and get some help. That's when I started those personal growth programs and hired coaches.

Today, I want to empower YOU to dedicate yourself to pursuing your healing. Then you'll make permanent shifts towards a better life. It works!

Today I have manifested a healthy, loving relationship. Manifested the love of my life, and together we're creating a very happy, loving, respectful family life. I am truly blessed.

**Jessica's last words:**

***"I had to be broken, to be rebuilt, to be the woman I am today" – Jessica DSB***

Turn your pain into power; also, be kind, be loving to yourself, and be compassionate with what you're feeling.

Always with love, Jessica DSB

# CHAPTER 6: Mind-Body Connection Healing

I strongly believe there is a real connection between the mind and body. We, as a whole, can be healed as a spiritual, emotional, and mental being. Now that I've learned more about integrative health and functional medicine, I can feel the gap between mental and physical treatment.

If someone has been diagnosed with depression, anxiety, and PTSD symptoms, chances are high that there could be other imbalances in their physical body. When we are in an acute condition and we need immediate help, like if we've broken our leg, had an asthma attack, a car crash, or any other physical health issues, we go to hospital. But with PTSD and mental health, we tend to wait until we have been properly diagnosed before we believe it is a genuine illness. Then most doctors medicate the patients with antidepressant drugs to subdue the symptoms and may suggest therapy or other calming solutions. That's only one side of the coin. If a doctor has experienced mind-body connection modalities, he/she may go deeper and refer the patient to someone who also checks him on a physical level.

Treating the symptoms only touches the surface; it may only give you a temporary relief. If the hidden layers don't have opportunities to be discovered, the symptoms will show up again at a later time.

During last year, I had around 200 interviews with health care practitioners, medical doctors, and holistic medicine practitioners, who all believed in mind-body connection and healing modalities. They talked about their patients and how they could treat depression by treating gut issues, weight-loss, healthy diets, exercise, and lifestyle changes.

In my fertility coaching practice I always make a full assessment of the body as a whole, not just their specific symptoms. I have discovered, there might be a bigger reason behind the PCOS or endometriosis. As mind and body are connected, I go deeper and look to see if the patients have physical symptoms of a chronic disease. I investigate their belief systems, and past trauma experiences, rather than just treating their physical body. That's the same when it comes to dealing with depression.

Personality disorder, despair, anxiety, eating disorder, Post-Traumatic Stress Disorder, or any mental health issues remain stored in our bodies at a cellular level for a long time. These may also cause hidden physical damage as well.

# Lise Leblanc - Registered Psychotherapist, Master Coach Practitioner, Clinical Hypnotherapist

Lise Leblanc is an author of 9 books, including *The PTSD Guide* and *PTSD Guide Workbook*. She uses cognitive behavior therapy in conjunction with hypnotherapy to treat clients with various issues, including PTSD.

She also has a personal history of childhood trauma and has undergone a huge intensive healing journey of her own. It helped her be a better therapist and understand what really works with treating trauma.

**PTSD Recovery by Creating a Strong Mind and Body Connection by Lise Leblanc**

PTSD creates functional and structural changes in the brain and nervous system. It also alters the way hormones and neurotransmitter's function. It's really important to understand this because even though PTSD has psychological aspects, the basis of it is in the nervous system.

This doesn't mean there is nothing we can do to change it; it just means we also have to work at the nervous system level. We can talk all day long about the traumatic event, but until we disarm some of those painful memories, they will continue to trigger our nervous system into fight-flight-freeze mode.

It's a vicious cycle. The amygdala becomes oversensitive (to protect us), activating the fear response, which then it floods the hippocampus with stress hormones, creating even more damage in the nervous system.

It is very important for people to understand this when you're dealing with PTSD. It's not a matter of just "dealing with it" or "thinking positive". Nor does it suggest that you just need to try harder.

This is very frustrating because it's not that simple when your brain and nervous system are not cooperating. It's not about trying harder. It's about releasing some of the painful emotions and the meanings attached to traumatic experiences. Then your nervous system can be trained to relax.

I went through a lot of childhood trauma, and I grew up being very fearful and anxious. As a teenager, I suffered from anxiety, depression, an eating disorder, substance abuse, and thoughts of suicide. I didn't know trauma was at the root of my problems.

I didn't want to deal with my trauma. I wanted to just pack it down, hold it down, and never look at it ever again. I tried to distract myself away from any of those traumatic thoughts and memories, but they were always running in the background of my mind and triggering my fear response.

As I went through my 20's I got increasingly anxious and depressed. I tried all the quick-fix solutions. By the time I was 30, I had a mental and emotional breakdown. I went to see my doctor, who gave me medication, but that didn't help much.

Therapy came next and it was helpful to talk about the things that had happened to me. But it didn't get to the root of my trauma. I started having other problems like irritable bowel syndrome, frequent infections, and some numbness in my hands and feet. My nervous system was going awry.

At that point in my life, I was working as a therapist and my main therapeutic approach was Cognitive Behaviour Therapy (CBT). CBT was extremely helpful for some clients, but I noticed it wasn't working that well with many of my clients with PTSD.

Even though they knew what they were "supposed" to do, they just couldn't change their thinking or their behaviour when triggered. In my case, my nervous system was so traumatized, CBT wasn't enough. I really had to dig deeper, and so I went on a huge healing journey.

I went to Peru and did ayahuasca ceremonies, then I hiked to the Grand Canyon. I went to retreats and read every self-help book I could get my hands on. Then I really dove in deep and did hypnotherapy. It created some deep subconscious shifts that helped me release and re-process some of the trauma that was trapped in my nervous system.

This healing experience got me onto this path of using hypnotherapy to help my clients reinterpret and release their traumatic memories and experiences. When bringing clients into such a deep relaxed state, into that parasympathetic state, it allows them to view their life experiences from a different psychological and physiological state.

They can review the timeline of their life from a calm, detached perspective and go back to those significant traumatic emotional events they've never had the chance to process, reinterpret, integrate, or release.

So, we go right into those experiences while in this ultra-relaxed state, and I guide them to release the emotion and the meaning attached to those traumatic experiences so that their nervous system can go back into relaxation and healing mode.

Hypnotherapy allows the person to go into the creative and emotional side of the brain and shift memories and emotions that are keeping their nervous system stuck. Many people believe that memories are like a video recording, but the fact is, we edit and modify memories all the time.

What I help people do is change certain memories in a way that allows them to release the emotion associated with them. Then they are able to put the memory back into storage in a way that's more tolerable. Then they are able to move forward in a way that allows their nervous system to repair itself.

## Lise's last Words

You can't heal what you can't feel, but you can't heal what you can't face, either. I think the biggest mistake for people who face trauma is to bury it. It's like having a knife stabbed into your leg and taking painkillers to distract yourself from the pain. You can forget about it for a while, but you're still bleeding out.

When I start working with someone new, I always begin with their trauma timeline. We start by facing what they've been through, looking at it and working on it consciously. Then, we get into the subconscious mind. It picks up anything associated with the trauma and amplifies it.

We need to de-activate those triggers, otherwise, more and more things get associated with the traumatic event and next thing, you're triggered almost constantly. When you're on that emotional side of your brain, there's no reasoning with it. It does not speak the same language; so, your rational mind might be using all the positive talk, but there's no connection between the rational and emotional sides of the brain.

It's really important to have strategies that work directly on your nervous system, like having a grounding kit ready with things that quickly bring you back into the now. It works to awaken your senses because your senses are communicating directly with your amygdala.

I tell my patients to have some sour candies or something that is positively associated with your childhood, things that immediately make you feel safe. These can be sights, sounds, smells that are already associated with safety and security.

Prepare yourself in advance because once triggered into fight-flight-freeze, it's no longer the time to make rational decisions and figure out what you need to do to feel better.

I hope that by understanding PTSD better, and what really works when it comes to treating trauma, will help you in your journey to healing.

# Jeannine L. Rashidi, Health and Wellness Practitioner

I had two interviewees in my shows about Ayurvedic medicine which originates from Hindu culture and is a holistic approach to healing. The concept is very similar to Chinese medicine. If you need more information, you can refer to the research study from the US National Library of Medicine to know the differences between these healing modalities[12].

Jeannine Rashidi is the author of *Abundance Beyond Trauma*[13], which was published in May 2021. She has been in the health and wellness industry now, for the last 18 years, which includes many forms of bodywork and trauma-informed mental and emotional integration work. She is an Ayurvedic practitioner and is in her last year of Ayurveda doctor training.

Jeannine's experience over 25-years of healing her own trauma and PTSD, her 18 years of experience, and the "I'm triggered! Pocket Guide" and the EDHIR ® Process that she created, helps many on their healing journey.

**Jeannine L. Rashidi' story, Confronting Triggers Through Ayurvedic Medicine by**

The name of my practice is 'Goodbye tension; physical, mental, emotional, and digestive relief". From an Ayurvedic perspective, the first thing we look at is your ability to digest not only in the gut but mentally and emotionally. There are foods and lifestyles that can increase the possibility of symptoms like anxiety, depression, and more. It all depends on one's current level of digestion mentally and physically.

In the first 25-years of my life, I suffered severely from physical, mental, emotional, psychological, and sexual abuse. My parents were very unhealthy, but when I was 15-years old—being a high-achieving student—I was lucky to be surrounded by teachers who were very supportive.

"Where are the classes that teach me how to deal with what's going on at home?" I remember asking them. They told me there weren't any. So, I decided it would be better if I ran away.

I hitchhiked 500-miles and learned how to live homeless with some of the Vietnam Vets. I didn't understand what PTSD was being only 15, but I learned how to relate with people who had triggers.

During that time, I met a man 17-years my senior who didn't intend to follow in his parents' footsteps of addiction and trauma. Unfortunately, that is exactly what ended up happening.

I left one abusive experience and went right into another for 10-years. But now, I had children. I gave birth to my first daughter when I was 16, and my second daughter at 20. I realized as time passed, they were exhibiting the same symptoms I had from my traumatic experience.

So, I started asking myself questions, like, how did this happen? I left home to get away from all that abuse, and I fell right back into that same cycle.

When you don't heal the pain from the trauma you experienced, statistics say you may fall into the exact same cycle of abuse, or, even worse, you may, without intention, become the abuser. I certainly didn't want my daughters to end up like me as pregnant teens in abusive relationships; I certainly didn't want them to become drug addicts.

So, I began my own healing practice purely with the intention of being able to survive and make money, while creating my own hours.

I no longer wanted to be a statistic, so when I could leave that situation with my daughters and start a new life, my first goal was to change that cycle of dysfunction and abuse. I learned about the Ayurvedic Perspective and found out I was really good at it. All the clients I saw had trauma. But I still questioned myself.

"Am I the right person for this?" I was somebody who was triggered all the time. "Can I help someone else when I'm still healing my own trauma?" Turns out the universe is very serendipitous that way, and it was the perfect profession for me.

When I started writing my book *Abundance Beyond Trauma,* I kept thinking about the one thing I wished I'd had when I was going through it. A cheat sheet, cheat code, or pocket guide to help me get out of that state.

So, I developed a process called "EDHIR ®". It helps you come back to the heart and mind connection. There's a disconnect that happens in trauma, where it was too much for our psyche to handle. So, we disconnect and then later, we suffer from triggers.

That disconnected part of you that occurred during your trauma, tries to get your attention by sparking off a trigger. After many years, I see that triggers are actually blessings, because they show us the problems that are already there. We just need to have the courage to listen to what our body and mind are saying.

This "EDHIR ®" process that I created is very similar to what Lisa Leblanc talked about. It's the ability to go in, explore and identify those parts of ourselves that are disconnected, that are showing up as a trigger.

When you look at yourself from a 360-degree perspective, you can see what you're lacking. The next step is to give that to yourself, like a guardian would.

Once healing has happened, you feel a sense of integration. That integration can happen through body work or through different visualization techniques. Once integration happens, you learn how to relate to yourself differently.

The pocket guide also includes the first three key factors for coming out of the trigger, which are:

1. When you're triggered, stop! Don't make any decisions. I assure you, it can have a tremendous impact on your life. Take a universal 'timeout' from your situation and catch your breath. It can be very difficult to take deep, slow breaths when adrenaline is pumping, especially when somebody tells you to. But if you concentrate on the flow of your inhales and exhales, you can get it under control. Start with two quick inhales and a long exhale. Follow that pattern until your breathing slows down.
2. Locate. During the fight, flight, or freeze response, the mind needs something to do to bring it back to a present state. The key is to keep your eyes moving so you don't freeze. Identify three objects around you. That will identify the time and space and bring you back to the present moment. Items like a plant, the cup of water beside you, or maybe the wind that's blowing in the trees. Again, keep following your breathing pattern throughout. Two quick inhales and one exhale.
3. Identify your well-wishers, the people you trust in your worst moments. Those you can reach out to who already know and understand what your trigger responses are. Thinking of them can bring the peace needed to step out of your triggered state. Stay with the breathing exercise throughout.

The rest of the steps to immediate relief from an activated state, are in the "EDHIR ®" process. The *"I'm Triggered! Pocket Guide"* are in the back of my book, *Abundance Beyond Trauma.* There's also a method that will heal that trigger.

## Jennine's last Words

My favorite phrase is the subtitle of my book:

*Discover your courage for change and commitment to yourself.*

# Dr Achina Stein, Osteopathic Physician, Functional Medicine Practitioner

Dr. Achina Stein is an osteopathic physician who graduated from UMDNJ School of Osteopathic Medicine in 1990. She has been in practice as a board-certified psychiatrist for 25-plus years. Her osteopathic roots set her apart from the conventional psychiatrists because of her use of osteopathic philosophy and the biopsychosocial treatment approach.

Initially, on a psychoanalytic track, she became well trained in psychodynamic psychotherapy and CBT. She does psychotherapy with a people who suffer with underlying trauma issues, specifically mood and dissociative disorders.

Dr. Stein has a wealth of experience using psychopharmacology with the prison population, community mental health centers, the persistent mental health population, geriatric psychiatry, and inpatient population. She understands the limitations of treatment with medication and is continually searching for other modalities of treatment.

Propelled by her son's health crisis in 2010, she found functional medicine, which resolved all his health problems and her own. Since then, Dr. Stein has been practicing functional medicine. She is certified by the American Board of Integrative and Holistic Medicine and is a certified practitioner of the Institute for Functional Medicine.

Dr. Stein is a Distinguished Fellow of the American Psychiatric Association and awarded the Exemplary Psychiatrist Award by NAMI-RI in 2008. Since 2012, she has been practicing functional medicine in her co-owned private practice in Rhode Island called *Functional Mind, LLC.*

From her experiences, she wrote a book called *What If It's Not Depression? Your Guide to Finding Answers and Solutions.* It's a guide to help you find the root causes of depression, which can be from foods, infections, toxins, and stress - all of which affect your hormones, especially the stress hormones.

You can work with her directly through her online health coaching program, *What If It's Not Depression?* Bootcamp. A 12-week system that assists you in reaching your health goals. She created it to help people find their root causes and bring their body back into balance. It ultimately resolves their depression without unnecessary medication.

**Dr Achina Stein' Story: PTSD, Gut, and Brain Connection**

A person with PTSD symptoms tends to be in 'fight-flight mode' or in 'sympathetic mode.' When this happens chronically—and particularly if it begins in childhood—their bodies surge with adrenaline. This then causes a surge of cortisol over long periods of time. It doesn't even have to be chronic. It could be a sudden change in stress or an acute stressor. A sudden stress can cause your gut to shut down.

Stress doesn't need to be psychological; it could be physical. A physical concussion can cause the gut to shut down, resulting in a host of problems. There is also a common connection with that, like having chronic anxiety due to an acute stressor—where you don't feel safe. Or wondering when the other shoe is going to drop, the walking-on-eggshells kind of anxiety. Triggers can cause chronic symptoms.

If you're in fear for your life, have a fear of danger, or are feeling very vulnerable, that can potentially cause 'leaky gut syndrome' or increased gut permeability. Our emotions affect our gut, and as a result, it can cause a whole host of symptoms. When you have increased gut permeability or 'leaky gut', sadly, that's just one of the issues.

The other issue is that your digestion system can shut down. This healing system, and your ability to rest, tends to shut down during sympathetic drive or fight-flight. You need to be in parasympathetic mode, which is the rest, digest, and heal mode, in order for digestion and sleep to occur.

A lot of times people have sleep problems when they have PTSD. That's very common, but when digestion shuts down too, you have difficulty releasing enzymes like pancreatic enzymes, hydrochloric acid, and bile salts which enable you to digest the carbs, the fats, and the proteins that you are eating.

If you're eating the right foods, you may not be digesting them and assimilating those nutrients into your body. Those are what enable you to handle your stress, so, over time, that can cause nutritional deficiencies and prevent you from managing stress in the long run.

The other complication is developing food sensitivities because of the increased (gut) permeability or leaky gut. It can also make you vulnerable to chronic gut infections. So, that's why a lot of people with PTSD get sick with different types of infections; yet another burden that your immune system needs to deal with.

Eighty percent of your immune system and neurotransmitters are made in the gut. When your gut isn't right, you can have a whole cascade of symptoms. A recently published article, "Gut-Brain Connection: Microbiome, Gut Barrier, and Environmental Sensors"[14] described how it is seen both ways, where changes to the gut lining can cause anxiety and stress symptoms.

If you can clean up and fix the gut, you can significantly improve not just anxiety and depression, but your entire health.

### Dr. Stein's last words

Don't give up. There is hope beyond medications and traditional psychotherapy.

# Dr. Manon Bolliger, Naturopathic Doctor and Founder of Bowen Therapy

After a few interviews with Dr. Manon Bolliger, I enrolled in the Bowen Therapy training. It's a mind-body reset course where you learn about her secrets behind her cancer and MS treatment. In her course, she emphasizes the need to listen to our body since nobody else can do it better than us.

Holistic medicine such as naturopathy, homeopathy, and acupuncture look at the whole body, mental and emotional state, and post-trauma disorders. Not just a regular diagnosis.

However, it's often difficult to share our deepest emotions with someone you really don't know. Some patients believe that it's an invasion of privacy. That's why they remain quiet about their emotional struggles and hidden layers of their chronic disease.

The first step in healing is self-care. The moment you realize you should prioritize your own health on top of everyone else's, even your own family members, your health improves. Nobody can carry your pain, even your loved ones, and nobody is responsible for your disease.

It's great to have support, but expecting everyone else to comfort you through entire process while you're complaining about your situation doesn't speed your healing journey. Unless you just believe in the power of healing and listen to your body and find all the imbalances within yourself.

I loved what Dr. Manon Bolliger said about her own healing journey:

***I can support myself by taking the time to reconnect to the sunrise and the moon and to stand on the grass and feel the earth.***

You are the creator of your life even if you have cancer or MS. Others may help you along the way, but healing starts when you feel peaceful inside and you care about your body, your emotions, and your recovery. We can retrain our brain and rewrite our story again.

Dr. Manon Bolliger is a Naturopathic doctor and CEO of Bowen College, TEDx speaker, the author of a best-selling book, *A Healer in Every Household,* and the host of "The Healers' café" podcast. She has been in practice for 30-years, and currently dedicates most of her time to running Bowen College, despite the limitations of the pandemic, where physical contact is not popular.

She believes, however, that it is extremely important to reset our physiology from the stress it has experienced. It's precious to anyone experiencing mental illness, PTSD, anxiety, or any emotional upset or issue. Even though touch is often overlooked, for Dr. Manon, it is a very important aspect to the entire integrated outlook on health.

**Dr. Manon Bolliger' stroy: The Correlation Between Trauma and Overall Health**

Everything that Dr. Stein said, I completely agree with. We are a holistic being and gut health is essential. So is the importance of rebalancing the parasympathetic system. It is foundational not just to deal with stress, but how it affects the way our body heals. We must get people out of this constant, exaggerated, sympathetic overdrive so the body can relax enough for all systems to function and heal.

We tend to miss the overall state of a person with PTSD, traumatic accidents, or chronic disease by breaking the body up into pieces. We have specialists catering to every single part but miss the whole.

It's not common in standard conventional medicine to look at disease holistically.

If a person has a car accident and develops whiplash, there is no point just working on the physical symptoms without addressing the trauma. That is why so many people have physiotherapy for years without ever having their autonomic nervous system recalibrated.

This is true whether the person has experienced a trauma, been injured, had nightmares about it, or someone they know has died. The spectrum of what's going on all at the same time is substantial. If we just go to see a psychologist for the emotions, or take tranquilizers and painkillers, we don't deal with, or rid ourselves of the trauma. If we just do body work thinking we're going to address the whiplash, there is a good chance we will not get anywhere.

You have to put Humpty-Dumpty back together again and see him as a whole being. In my experience, I have seen the biggest results when I include the context of the pain or trauma in their body. It is necessary to address the parasympathetic, the part of the autonomic nervous system that brings balance to the sympathetic nerves. The body will know it's safe to heal and reboot the body and the mind.

**Dr Manon Bolliger's last words:**

You are not broken, and you can heal.

# Debera Jensen, Childhood Trauma and Chronic Disease

Maybe you were that little boy who was hiding in a closet to protect yourself from your parent's fight, or a toddler girl who was neglected and abandoned. Now you have moved on with your life but suddenly you're diagnosed with a chronic disease and find yourself on a mission to discover the root cause.

Debera Jensen is a Rapid Relief Energy, Mindset, and Belief healer. She has had her own center for over 30-years. Now all her work is done virtually.

She originally got into trauma work because of her own experiences. A devastating car accident left her with a head injury and other major injuries. When the doctors all gave up on her, she went out in search of the answers for herself. She ended up finding brain integrations that helped her brain to come back, and then she had to overcome the trauma, the loss, the depression, and the anxiety. After coming out the other side of her challenges, she started a center to help others.

It was one thing to overcome her injuries from that accident, but then she discovered that years earlier, she had suffered from childhood trauma. It was buried deep in her subconscious mind. She had suffered most from the words and behaviors of her mother at an early age. For instance, she was an unwanted child to her mother, so it was clear throughout the years that things were not right.

Debera developed beliefs and impressions she had to change. Things like she didn't have value, wasn't listened to, wasn't heard or seen, and she wasn't enough. As you can well imagine, having those basic, negative underlying beliefs left her feeling unsupported and wondering why her life was not working.

But when she finally discovered how to release negative emotions and install positive beliefs that supported her (amongst other things) her life radically changed for the better. Now she helps other people to do the same — to conquer the trauma and to live the lives they wished they'd had all along!

## How to Cush Childhood Trauma

The first thing I do is to teach is how to leave self-sabotage behind. As long as that is in the way, it will prevent us from getting accurate answers on the help that is needed.

I also tap into my awareness. I am extremely intuitive, so I help find the negative beliefs buried in my patient's subconscious. Those perspectives negatively impact their behaviors and affects their life.

Then I help them to diffuse the negative emotions they received during their childhood and instill the positive beliefs which will support their life. Old, negative patterns are broken so new joyful patterns can turn everything around.

I also add daily brain integrations so they can leave the stress behind and feel better. This usually occurs within the first 1-2 hours. They know these processes are working because they feel the difference early on.[15]

# CHAPTER 7: First Responders' PTSD Prevention and Treatment

Imagine working in a demanding environment that needs your constant and immediate support. Where those referred to you are on the edge, deciding between life and death, and you need to respond quickly in order to save their lives. Working this type of job, being responsible for the welfare of others for 8-hours a day, may teach you how to act confidently when managing these acute conditions. But it exhausts your body and drains you mentally and emotionally long term.

I remember when my mother worked in an emergency room as a nurse. Her morning started with patients with acute conditions: a sudden stroke, car crash, hiking accident (since she used to work in a mountainous area), or any other unexpected accident.

She was the first one who gave us the news at home about any weird and deadly mishap in our region. Working as a first responder over long periods of time trains you to react quickly in emergency situations, but that go-go personality also affects your daily life.

One day, I and my three brothers were breaking and eating some roasted nuts. My mom came in from work and saw my youngest brother choking on them. She immediately held him from behind and delivered firm blows between his shoulder blades to help dislodge the nut's stuck in his throat.

Personally, I was shocked and couldn't move to help, but my mother took control of the situation and saved my brother's life without wasting her time and energy panicking. She is always calm and responsive in managing acute situations. After a while, her health declined, so she switched to a calmer hospital ward with a less stressed-out environment.

Recently I watched two wonderful series on Netflix about the life of Medical First Responders. *New Amsterdam* and *Chicago Med* are both great movies to show how these types of people sacrifice their own comfort for the sake of saving others.

The most important similarities in both series were the psychiatrists who attended any acute cases, supporting patients to find out the mental and emotional root-cause of the problem accompanying their physical disease or injuries.

Modern medicine now understands the importance of mind-body connection and why patients need emotional and mental support while treating their physical problems. Both series highlight the connection that PTSD has with hidden layers of some diseases. They give a sneak peek into first responders' personal lives, their own struggles with mental and physical health, and how their type of jobs have affected their families and romantic life.

I am grateful for the medical staff's continuous bravery and dedicated support during the pandemic. I believe now I understand their roles, their vulnerabilities, the nature of their jobs, and how to support them individually or as a part of our family.

I have interviewed three first responders in my different shows. Dr. Defne Neyman[16] who has worked as an emergency physician for over 25-years. Dr. Sajel Bellon[17], Psychotherapist, Professor, and TEDx Speaker who lived with a fire fighter husband. And Jason Coulthard, former Homicide and International Organized Crime Enforcement Detective with the Toronto Police. I've included Jason's interview in this book, so you can become familiar with what first responders do to confront PTSD.

# Jason Coulthard, International Organized Crime Enforcement Detective

Jason is a father of three daughters, 18, 16, and 14. He is the former Homicide and International Organized Crime Enforcement Detective with the Toronto Police.

In 1996, He started his career working as a uniform and plain-clothes officer at 52 Division, in the downtown core of Toronto. For 9-years, he worked as a Primary Response Officer, and a Community Response Officer, responding to calls for 9-1-1. He investigated street level drugs, breaking, and entering, and robberies for three years in the Major Crimes Unit.

As a community uniform officer, Jason was assigned to the Church Wellesley area, and took part in numerous demonstrations and riots, including the G20, the Queens Park Riots, and the firebombing of the US Embassy, both in uniform and plain clothes capacity.

In 2005, Jason started his 8-year stint as an International Organized Crime Detective in The Major Projects Section of the Drug Squad. During this time, Jason investigated organized crime groups from around the world who were involved in the importation of illegal commodities into the Greater Toronto area. They included heroin, cocaine, ephedrine, money, weapons, nuclear weapons, and human trafficking.

Jason's investigations touched Iran, Iraq, Afghanistan, Turkey, India, China, United States, and Australia, to name a few.[18]

Jason became a police officer to ensure that what happened to him when he was 10-years old would not happen to anyone else. Jason had suffered sexual assault.

In May 2017, when Jason was in his 21st year with the Toronto Police, and his third year as a Homicide Detective, everything that he'd experienced became too much. Jason took sick leave and was shortly after formally diagnosed with Post-Traumatic Stress Disorder, Major Depressive Disorder, Panic Disorder, and anxiety disorder. Prior to that, he had suffered 3-years of panic attacks while being medicated by the currently insured mental healthcare system.

In December 2017, Jason attended a retreat called *Be in Health,* where he found the truth about his injuries. He was healed of all prior symptoms because of this miraculous experience. Unfortunately, on December 22, Jason's psychiatrist would not believe he was healed. Not only that, but he was also forcibly locked up in a psychiatric unit for 21-days. Jason was essentially kidnapped, confined, and forced to let them administer noxious substances. He was told he would not be released unless he took the 'medication'.

After a very traumatic and educational 21-days inside the belly of the beast, Jason was released. As part of his healing, Jason put together traumatic timelines to identify moments in his life that impacted him. The original timeline started at conception and continued through to his career as a police officer. He had 54 items on his list.

Then Jason made another traumatic timeline specifically for what happened to him in the hospital. He ended up with 78 new traumatic events.

Because of this and many other experiences in Jason's life, including not being provided with the proper resources to heal from his mental health injuries, Jason gathered like-minded people around him. They are working towards bringing attention and change to the current insured mental healthcare system in Canada.

In 2020, Jason formed a national not-for-profit called New Hope - Field of Dreams that looks closer at these problems. He provides multitude natural solutions that when combined, promote the healing of operational stress Injuries, and help prevent them from returning.

To accomplish this, Jason is forming a team that will present a 12-part "Docuseries of Truth that will explore the ripple effect on Canada's front-line workers, who Jason calls Local Heroes.

The docuseries team will first interview military veterans, police officers, paramedics, firefighters, community housing officers, dispatchers, nurses, doctors, psychiatrists, social Workers, victim services, personal service workers, medical service workers, psychotherapists, psychologists, hospital security, court officers, Crown attorneys, corrections officers, morgue attendants, and autopsy technicians.

He wants to hear their perspectives. Then Jason's team will interview those who are most vulnerable and call for assistance when they are in a mental health crisis: children, parents, homeless, addicts, and those who have lost loved ones to overdose and suicide.

While doing this, Jason is also looking to provide solutions for the current mental health and opioid overdose, suicide crisis. To accomplish this, Jason has also put together a plan to build Family Revival Retreats in every community across Canada called New Hope Field of Dreams–Family Revival Retreats. The first goal is to heal the Local Heroes and their families.

These Retreats will be self-sustained, natural environments that provide a multitude of natural, renewable resources to address the underlying signs, symptoms, and syndromes that cause diseases in our lives.

Canada's first New Hope Field of Dreams–Family Revival Retreat is proposed to be located on 133-acres of land in Cambrai, Ontario. Jason continues to bring together local community resources in the Kawartha area of Ontario so they can work as one family to accomplish this goal.

Jason has formed partnerships with local community resources such as Heaven's Gait Ranch, Produce for Heroes, Habitat for Humanity,

Endeavour Centre, Veteran Farmers, Veteran Revival Retreats, Veterans Channel TV, Be in Health, Veterans House, Circle Organic, as well as students and faculty from Fleming College and Durham College.

New Hope Field of Dreams–Family Revival Retreat will apply the multi-pronged approach to address the underlying causes of Complex Post-Traumatic Stress Disorder. With the assistance of proven resources, properly trained mental health trauma practitioners will look into various physical signs, symptoms, syndromes, and diseases that manifest in our bodies.

They will provide an integrated healing approach that will filter and fuel our entire Triune Being, our spirit, soul, and body. They will provide resources that help prevent these injuries from returning.

Some of the natural, renewable resources being brought together are peer-to-peer support, equine therapy, canine therapy, art therapy in its many forms, and mobility therapy that will combine positive pathways of thought to assist with the repair of physical injuries. Other options are conservation activities, homesteading, eco therapy, being in touch with earth, wind, fire, and water, including revival pathways that will have several mentor stations to assist their overcomers with their pathway towards recovery.

Proper nutrition is also essential in providing the optimal health. To assist with this, they plan to build greenhouses to grow all the fruits, vegetables, and plants that you need to fuel your body.

To keep in line with a holistic remedy, New Hope Field of Dreams is also bringing together holistic practitioners, including naturopaths and nutritionists and their remedies. They are also concerned with the environment and habitat in and around these Family Revival Retreats.

They are taking slow, methodical steps to ensure that everything they do improves the carbon footprint and enhances the current natural habitat. Like turtle or butterfly sanctuaries, an apiary, and a fishery. They will have eco-enhancing processes such as ecosystem management, ecological restoration, regenerative agriculture, sustainable agriculture, aqua farming, ecological farming, arboriculture, permaculture, culinary biodiversity, and animal biodiversity conservation.

To assist with becoming a self-sustainable environment, New Hope Field of Dreams is exploring regenerative power and natural building processes. They are researching geothermal energy, hydroelectricity, solar water purification, concentrated solar power, solar thermal energy, electro-magnetic induction, bioenergy, as well as rainwater harvesting, repurposing, hempcrete, and straw bale construction.

To do this, they're gathering local community resources. They're not reinventing the wheel. Instead, they are reaching out to organizations who are already self-sustainable and asking them to take part.

Their goal for 2022 is to work with our front-line services and Habitat for Humanity to facilitate team building and peer-to-peer support days to assist with the construction of the retreat.

They are bringing together various teams from police, fire, paramedic, nurses, and other Local Heroes to learn about New Hope Field of Dreams and their various processes of healing not just for one another, but also for the environment.

**Jason Coulthard's story: Confronting Triggers by Creating Environmental Awareness as a First Responder**

I have very minimal triggers now. Before they were abundant all the time. I had to go back into my traumas to deal with them. As a police officer and a lot of times as a child, you're not allowed to experience your thoughts and your emotions; so essentially, you write them down on a rock or a boulder; you throw them in your backpack, and you carry on with life. Then suddenly, signs and symptoms develop.

We get sick and get into a state of disease. I had to recognize a lot of things in my environment. What is my environment? Like you, it's my eyes, ears, nose, and mouth. Our environments are quite expansive. I had to recognize those things that caused me to trigger. The sounds, senses, sights, and vibrations. Perhaps you'll need to go even deeper and explore the energy side.

It's crucial to be very aware of your environment. We are spiritual beings. We have a soul that is full of our experiences, made up of our mind, will, and emotions. We live in a motor home, which is our body, which comprises of our brain, our heart, and our gut. Our spirit is made from the Father, the Son, and the Holy Spirit, and again our soul is formed from our mind, will, and emotions.

When we filter and fuel all nine areas correctly and we are aligned with the truth and true love, we are in our best, overall, optimal health. We must ensure that we lead a healthy lifestyle, which includes proper nutrition, being careful about what we're listening to and watching. We need to have the right people in our environment. A family who cares about you and loves you for who you are. People who want to empower you to become a better person, to uncover your traumatic triggers and replace them with truth and love. Those who will always be there for you.

As a coach, it is imperative that I am aware of various responses to emotional trauma. Such as the Three F's - Fight, Flight, and Freeze. When you are a peer-to-peer support person, you have to be able to hold a safe space for whoever is going through that traumatic trigger event. To help them walk through it with love, compassion, and understanding. You need to be able to feel to heal.

When a life coach or mentor is providing a safe space for someone to overcome their trauma, they also have to be aware of the transfer of energy or spirits when proper healing is applied.

Without that knowledge of the spiritual realm, a life coach or a mentor can become consumed with other people's traumas. There can also be some major generational blockages that prevent healing from manifesting.

The number one reason someone is not healing is unforgiveness. Being aware of the presence of entities or energies that are unseen by the naked eye is a huge part of recognizing the cause and effect. It is also imperative to have an in-depth knowledge about the generational causes of diseases that are passed down through generations. These include heart disease, cancer, sexual perversion, low self-esteem, mental health injuries, and suicidal tendencies.

In order to get rid of your triggers, you must look inside and upward in order to see things from a different perspective. As a first responder going into certain situations, we see what we see, as we have one set of eyes. Each event has many perspectives.

As an organized crime detective, I didn't just take one person's information accurately. To prove the evidence in our current courts of law, I had to investigate all areas of the evidence. Then eventually, I had an impartial, in-depth, and introspective view of the situation which allowed me to find accurate truth.

Another way I have repaired from my past trauma is recognizing and breaking soul ties. Soul ties can manifest into 3D images, flashbacks, nightmares, intrusive, negative, and destructive thoughts. These need to be dealt with to heal you from your past traumas.

I do this through meditation and prayer. As mentioned, I was sexually assaulted when I was 10-years old. I learned I detached from my traumatic event. Meaning that my soul was removed in that moment based on what I had experienced.

I have seen the traumatic events from these very impactful perspectives, including my sexual assault as a young child, and it brought about 100% healing. If I ever saw my aggressor, I would look him right in the eyes and tell him: "I forgive you; I love you, and I can't believe what you went through." Then I'd give him a hug. That's where I stand right now, how far I've come.

I am 48-years old and for 35-years; I held on to all these emotions. Currently, I am going through a divorce and my body is reacting to the emotions that I am experiencing as I go through this as well.

Specifically, I have been experiencing symptoms of irritable bowel syndrome. Because of all the strife in my relationship, I have been holding on to a lot of guilt, shame, and false burden bearing. The separation has also caused me to feel unloved, rejected, unwanted, and insecure in myself. That's resulted in me not loving or accepting myself, rejecting who I am now, and not letting go of who I was in the past.

My symptoms manifested after experiencing a traumatic event at work. I attended a car accident alone as a police officer and there were so many people injured. There was no way I could possibly save everyone, not even the child in the back of the car. Shortly after, as the days progressed, I remember having irritable bowel syndrome.

Recognizing your emotions and thoughts from a different perspective is how I've healed from trauma. It has not been an easy journey by any means. As a 'tough guy' with a badge and a gun, in uniform or out, we were not encouraged to feel our emotions, or express our thoughts.

However, as I have mentioned, to heal, you must feel. I have cried more over the past 3 ½ years of my recovery than I have in my entire life. This has been essential to my healing. Experiencing my emotions in a safe non-judgemental environment, and then picking myself back up off the ground, helped me feel lighter every time. I see it as crushing one rock at a time and building a new ladder-of-life got me out of my trauma hole.

As a police officer, I followed the rules that were given to me. I followed the mental health act, which gave me the freedom to use as much force as necessary to either arrest people when they're a danger to themselves or to others. Also, for those who couldn't take care of themselves.

I was mandated to take them to a safe place, which is a psychiatric unit. Then I was kidnapped and locked inside of one them for 21-days myself and administered noxious substances. I know what happens inside those hospitals. That's the reason people don't want to go.

Being a police officer can be terrible. You have people threatening suicide, others are physically cutting themselves. I don't want to go into too much detail with my experiences, but it's all a lot to deal with. When you are in those circumstances, you must make decisions and follow the rules.

I had one event where a fellow on the fifth floor of a building threatened to jump off the balcony. My partner and I ended up apprehending him under the mental health act and transported him safely to the hospital to get help.

I went back to the station and while I'm writing my report, there was a call for a male being stabbed in the face in the same apartment.

The male that we took to the hospital to be assessed, left the hospital, and went back and stabbed his boyfriend in the face. Apparently, the hospital found no grounds to keep him there. Yet they held me for 21-days. This is a problem that doesn't make sense.

I would do things differently now because I understand mental illness. I understand psychosis, schizophrenia; I understand double mindedness and detachment. I've gone through and continue to go through those things regularly.

My spiritual eyes have been opened. I see things from a very different perspective. Now, I help the less fortunate, the homeless people in Oshawa. In my newfound experiences, through a different lens, and from a totally unique perspective, I see how a lot of the homeless or less fortunate people are spiritually enlightened.

Not to say their pathways of thought are correct all the time, but they see, feel, and hear things that others don't. For example, I get transcending body pains in my body that show me where people's injuries are in their body. I've stood in front of somebody with emphysema and suddenly, my chest gets tight, and I can't breathe well.

I ask the person who came into my environment what was going on in their chest, and I was told COPD and emphysema. Then I was led in my spirit to lay hands on the man. I experienced and continue to experience this transfer of energy and the power of Jesus.

I prayed for his healing and asked in the name of Jesus for our Heavenly Father to reverse all damage the enemy has caused. Then I demanded that all generational curses put upon him that deal with the fear of abandonment, the spirit of death, or any orphan spirits to come out in the name of Jesus. I also asked that every proton, neutron, and electron to be formed back in the fearful and wonderful image of the Father, Son, and the Holy Spirit. I commanded all airways to be opened and any blockages be removed with the blood of Jesus.

In that moment, my chest expanded, his chest expanded, and we could both breathe again. God allowed this man to be healed from his COPD and emphysema. I also felt led to tell him the recent passing of his wife was not his fault and that God called her to come home. There was nothing that he could have done differently that would have prevented her from going home to God. He cried deeply and was released of any shame, guilt, abandonment, or fear of blame and was healed by God.

We are all connected, and we need to love one another as brothers and sisters and to forgive one another. Our battles are not with the flesh and blood of this world, nor are they with each other.

Our battles are with spiritual entities of unseen places and rulers of dark kingdoms. You are not a bad person. If you just did a bad thing, recognize it. Forgive yourself and others for all the negative thoughts and emotions that have been causing you emotional trauma for so long.

As a human race, we're all one family and it's through love, empathy, understanding, caring, and compassion, we can heal one another. Giving people a safe space to just be, allowing them to be around people like yourselves, who have a deeper understanding of trauma, is the best way to heal.

This is what I needed in 2001 when my PTSD started. I consumed what the world was offering me, the pills, alcohol, porn, and improper use and abuse of marijuana.

I needed to be surrounded by like-minded, holistic people, not doctors and psychiatrists who threw me a bunch of pills and told me to come back in six weeks. This was torturous.

***If you want to torture someone,***

***give them PTSD without a solution.***

There are solutions, there is hope. But it's time for a change!

I will continue to bring groups of like-minded people from across Ontario and across Canada together to gain a deeper understanding of what trauma is, why it happens, and how to fix your trauma.

I will teach them how to filter and fuel their entire Triune Being—spirit, body, and soul—with the truth, to obtain overall optimal health. To get back to the roots of creation, to move from a place of barely surviving life to thriving.

**Jason's last words:**

You have the power inside of you to heal. Greater is he that lives inside of you than he that is in the world. Take what the enemy meant for evil and turn it into good. Recognize the rocks from the past you're carrying. Crush them and then build a ladder to get you out of the hole you're in. Lose your pride. ***YOU NEED TO FEEL TO HEAL.***

One Love, Jason Coulthard

# CHAPTER 8: How to Rewrite Your Life's Story and Rejoice After Being Hit by Trauma

I was looking at a short documentary about an eagle trying to fly after years of being kept in the cage. She was standing on the top of the mountain and looking down the hill, scared and hesitant to fly. It was so sad to see how such a powerful bird, with a heavy head and beak, a bird that flies higher than others, was now too captivated by her thoughts that she couldn't open her wings.

It took some time for her to realize she was a bird in nature, and she only needed to remember how to fly. Then she opened her wings a few times and finally overcame her fears. She took off so high into sky; it was breathtaking.

How many of us have forgotten how to fly? Dare we release the chains of our limited beliefs, open our wings, and fly?

We are all born with unique talents and exclusive abilities, but only those who believe in their powers can overcome their fears and fly to the full height of their potential. PTSD can substitute our strength with fear and paralyze us from any positive movement.

We may prefer to stay in our comfort zone and let ourselves be manipulated by our thoughts and past traumas. On the other hand, we can pull ourselves out of the darkness and enter a bright future by retraining our brain and rebuilding our best life.

While learning how to knit, sometimes I had to pull and undo the entire row even if there was only one flawed stitch. Every event, an emotional breakdown, or trauma, whatever led to PTSD, needs to be looked at and processed to stop it from affecting your future.

I went through a transition every time I was knocked down, but I rose again. I discovered it's difficult to start over while still needing time to heal. Or to be ready for our next move when trauma is more severe. Some events take longer to be fully understood and processed.

In chapter 6 of my third book *Naturally Conceived,* I talked about a formula which always helps me speed up the process to get back on track. I call it PAUSE:

P- Pause

A - Adjust

U - Unite

S - Surrender

E - Educate.

We all need a break to learn where we are standing and how we would like to move forward. What we do during the gap can be crucial for building or ruining our future.

Let's have a quick sneak peek at that formula.

1. **Pause:** when I am overwhelmed with emotional burdens, I pause and stop all other necessary tasks and avoid over-analysing my situation. After being hit by a sudden trauma, you may need more time to pause. I always recommend my fertility patients to pause at least for 3-4 months. In other cases, that may vary depending on your readiness and severity of PTSD. Put a halt to

the daily noises. It is a great time to accept your situation, find more peace and tranquility.

2. **Adjust:** As soon as you are ready to move on, you may find ways to not only adapt to your new situation after loss, accident, or any other traumas, but you may also need to check out your physical, mental, and emotional condition. Balancing your mental health may need you to look at your lifestyle, your physical health, and even balancing your hormones. That's what you call self-care. Body, spirit, and mind as a whole, should be taken care of when you are trying to adapt to a new situation. Ask yourself, "Where are you, and where do you wish to be? What do you need to change in order to feel more peaceful and resume your life again?" Maybe you need to make new connections, study a new course, or relocate to another place. You can transform into the new you with better planning and a willing heart.
3. **Unite:** If you have a considerate partner, a close friend, or a fellow family member, team up as accountability partners. The reason behind it is to have someone trustworthy to rely on; someone who loves to see you feel better, happier, and healthier. I love support groups. Whatever I wish to learn, I join the support group; a community of like-minded people who follow the same target, have the same challenges, and inspire each other to become stronger. When I republished my first book, I teamed up with an accountability partner who also wanted to write her book. We shared our experiences along the way and set up a weekly plan to achieve our goals faster. There are so many people with bright ideas who wish to be an author, but their inspiration declines over time. That's the same with PTSD recovery or any healing process. Having an accountability partner is helpful to keep you on track and push you toward your ideal target.
4. **Surrender:** You may have heard people say that they just surrendered, and it happened. This is especially true for couples who have been struggling with infertility for a long time. Surrender

means to yield to the power of divinity. It ensures that a greater source of energy leads you to a higher level of being. Then, you need to stop over-analyzing and enjoy your life while you are in the healing process.

5. **Educate:** Knowledge is power. While struggling with my PTSD, I started my self-development journey by reading empowering books and continuing my study in Australia. Trauma can mess up your life, but it can also teach you some essential lessons and create new opportunities to see the world from a different perspective. It's also a great distraction to stop overthinking and help focus your energy on something more interesting than worrying and envisioning your past trauma. That doesn't mean to totally ignore what has happened, but it's a great tool to boost your confidence and retrain your brain. Then you may need to find some other tools like NLP (Neuro-Linguistic Programming) and hypnotherapy; it can help process your hidden layers of PTSD and change your perception about different areas of your past trauma.

I have also written about four stages of creating sustainable change in my first book, *Rules of Change for the Better.*

# Debbie Pace. Energy Healer

One of the big things Debbie does is to help people work with their own energy to heal their trauma. She highly recommends people to practice good  breathing. That is the best place to start when looking to get out of any trauma response you find yourself in.

**Rewrite Your Life: Debbie Pace Story**

I experienced some deep childhood trauma growing up with a violent father in the first few years of my life. There were a lot of things wired into my brain, and as a result, I was in a fight-or-flight response my entire life. It affected everything, especially my personal relationships.

My husband and I married in 2004, but it ended in divorced. However, through some massive inner work I did, I could reconcile our marriage in less than two years.

Now I help others to use the breathing to pause their trauma responses. Once we've calmed down the nervous system, we go in and look at where the stories in their head are coming from, and then we work on rewriting them and rewiring them into their physical and mental bodies.

A lot of what I do going deep into where the trauma lies and where the stories and beliefs stem from. Then I have them take ownership of their own story. In a nutshell, you make your story come from inside you instead of from the original source that came from outside of yourself.

**Debbie Pace's Solution**

What I do - not only in my own life but in what I teach clients too - is really just taking responsibility for how we show up in life. It is very important to remember and understand that you're no longer in the trauma, you're no longer in the situation that caused pain. You are safe.

So, first, focus on your breathing and it will settle down the trauma response and help you reconnect to your true inner self. Then, you take responsibility and take action by writing down what you really want your life to look like.

You can ask yourself questions like:

"How do I want to show up now?" "How do I want to feel now?" "Who do I want to be now?"

It takes a conscious effort every single day. I also incorporate other healing modalities, such as sound healing and Reiki. I'm also a certified practitioner of a process called Quantum Flow, which works with the physical body to basically rewire all the outdated stories and physiological responses stored within our physical and energetic bodies. It does this from the inside out.

I spent four decades of being plugged into that trauma, so every single day it requires the physical, emotional, and spiritual work to get that out of my system. Then I get to be the person who's no longer in that trauma, but one who is living life on purpose and in joy.

# Part 2

## Expert Chapters

My sincere thanks to Richard Morden, Roseline Salazar, Maricelly Ramos, Linda Hays Cooper and Nancy Nance for contributing to these chapters. Thank you for sharing your own personal stories of overcoming grief, combatting PTSD, domestic violence, abusive relationships, and living gracefully with ADHD. This part mostly focuses on solutions and antidotes.

# CHAPTER 9: I Cannot Understand Normal Thinking by Nancy Nance

My truth is that I lived in a house of horrors that held a dark secret. Homes are built on solid foundations that keep what we value secure. Each wall keeps the danger out and the love in. Carefully constructed rooms are built to house the sweet love we've vowed to protect. It is within those walls that secrets are kept. But not all secrets are meant to remain hidden.

As I tell you my secrets, I no longer cower in the corner, afraid to share my shame. Shame no longer holds me captive. Guilt no longer governs my actions. Courage helps me hold my sword strong. Strength is how I keep walking when I am tired. Faith allows me to move forward through the forest that is often so dark. Grace shines her light on every challenge so I can see the opportunities before me. The light of love is what I use to show me which path to follow.

Following fear kept me in the catacombs where women are kept in abuse. Abuse is how hurt people continue to hurt. Hurt opens the door to healing. Hurt is my story, and healing is my mission. My mission is also to help heal the world of hurt. I began with my own hurts. I owned each one and found solutions I can now share with you. The process of healing I used is now the process I share to shine a light for those who are ready to begin.

Some stories don't have endings. With each new sunrise, another chapter of our life is opened. The sun rises to welcome the day so we can continue our journey to our predestined purpose. The purpose of life is to live in joy, embrace peace, and create a life worth living.

My life wasn't always worth living. I was trapped in a lie for 25-years and I didn't leave my lie. My lie left me.

"I love you, but I'm not in love with you," were the most shocking words I'd heard our entire marriage. It was an autumn evening when my ex-husband told me those words.

"No shit, Sherlock," I said. "I haven't loved you for years." Now I know I only stayed so one day, I could escape my marriage and go to university with my daughter. For 15-years I planned my escape. I had every piece of the puzzle in place except one. How was I going to make it all work when I knew the liar wouldn't let me leave.

I hid the truth from absolutely everyone beneath a mountain of lies. Or so I thought. I believed I had to keep the truth hidden or it would ruin our lives. There was no other option. I was able to create an escape plan, pretend that all was well, even though it was all falling apart. Every stitch of the seams of my life were bursting apart one at a time.

Later, I found out that everyone knew, and yet no one helped. Battalions of blame surrounded my existence, and I didn't know how to fight. I had learned that fighting brought me pain, so I put on a fake smile, faced the music, and made the best of things.

The 'best of things' were my children. We lived an idyllic life with family vacations, and fancy houses, but we were drowning in a sea of debt, and the life raft had floated away, far out of reach. I found myself separated from the lifeboats of family, friends, and faith. But I kept a fake smile on my face.

Monsters are scary and my monster knew how to erect walls around me to keep me separated from all forms of rescue. My monster was the father of my children and the man I vowed to live with until death do us part.

Death split our family into a million little pieces. I couldn't keep my marriage together and do the one thing I was counselled to do. Take care of myself. Sounds simple, except I struggled because they also expected me to keep my monster happy. If only I had seen the truth earlier, I would have chosen a different life. I would not have married the man who ruined mine. I would have become a teacher, built a peaceful home, had five fabulous children, two dogs, and a cat. But that's not the life I chose.

Signing that marriage certificate led to a life filled with domestic violence, greed, drugs, whiskey, and whores. I became everything I despised as I tried to navigate the darkest depths of hell. Every part of me that was sweet became bitter.

Later in my future, I took that bitterness and transformed it into gold. I chipped away at the pain until my heart was healed.

But back then, I had to become a chip off the old block and embrace my inner bitch. Being a bitch was easier than being a battered woman. So, I embraced my bad attitude and learned the fine art of creative writing.

I was inspired by the people I trusted. The ones who knew the truth about my life. There were few, but they were fierce. They knew the tangled web I'd woven and understood that in order to unravel it, I would have to become bold, braver, more bad-ass version of myself.

They cheered as I began writing my truth. I became a B-I-T-C-H (Babe in Total Control of Herself) and loved the power it gave me. I poured anger out of each open wound in my life. What normally destroys lived, I survived. I took each trauma, terror, and form of treachery he conducted and used them to navigate my boat on the sea of uncertainty.

I used my potty-mouth and my shitty-attitude as I stepped into the unknown abyss of divorce. The problem is, I trusted the only person in my life whose voice I had listened to.

My ex-husband offered me the deal of a lifetime and I took it hook, line, and sinker. I built a new life in a new home and believed that all the hurt could be healed with a piece of paper. That lavish deal was a lie, and I learned quickly how cruel the courts could be. I had no idea that what was rightfully mine, that justice I deserved, would be withheld. That cocaine and crack would once again steal my calm and destroy my home.

The truth is, I'm not always Nice-Nancy who only speaks when she is spoken to. I am not the perfect daughter who is dutifully seen but not heard. I am not the gracious ghost who keeps the family secrets hidden in the dark. I am much more than that.

Truth is, I am a pretty book of words that are not meant to be spoken. I am a C-U-N-T for I Cannot Understand Normal Thinking. Normal is not the life I lived before my divorce.

I dissected 25-years of 'not normal' and healed every whispered weakness and perceived threat. I battled for my healing within the sacred shallows of my mind. I invited every ghostly memory, triggered trauma, and manic moment in the dark dance where healing takes place.

The final straw came with my divorce. As my ex-husband pulled the pin on his threat, I placed the grenade in my mouth and swallowed. Never again would I text him, speak to him, or play his game. He told me to collect the money he owed me from my son, his son, the son whose life he'd ruined. The same son who came to learn that forgiveness is the path that leads to love.

Forgiveness leads to the promised land where we learn to forgive ourselves. I allowed my son to walk his path as I walked my own. Together, we discovered everything would be provided to us if we did the work. So, we worked hard and found the justice we deserved. We put on our shields, held our swords high, and with strength, we pursued justice. We readied ourselves for the battle we were determined to win. I was ready, willing, and waiting to see what would happen next.

God brought me my lawyer through LegalShield and an amazing group of ladies. They're not your typical ladies and he's not your typical lawyer. He wasn't my first choice, but Mister Horne was more than I expected. I am grateful for his tact.

When I don't have the know-it-all, I know when to add a player to my team. He drives the legal car when I need to win a race. That road was long, but I had plenty of gas in my tank. My Ladies of Justice helped me when things got tough, and sometimes times still get tough.

Together, we worked on creating a stew to serve him and when the perfect opportunity came, the angels helped me serve the demand letter.

I began the delivery process in December when 20/20 vision obscured most people's lives behind a mask. Three failed attempts in six months were followed by a stint in rehab. He had once again promised to get clean, and I allowed my lawyer to use the chance to try again.

Quitters never win and winners never quit. We tried again, and he tried for the fourth time in another drug rehabilitation centre. Hope led me to believe he had surrendered to his healing. I believe everything is possible when you call upon God and have the courage to change.

I have written about the courage it took to heal in several books, with fabulous friends, for amazing, and just causes. *Helping Sacred Heart Rise* was an honour I authored twice.

I am truly blessed with the many opportunities it has given me to heal. Each time my pen takes me on a journey, I pray God will help me once again understand serenity. Each lesson learned is a penny earned in my karmic bank account.

The Law of Cause and Effect was brought to earth to help us all govern our actions. The consequences of my choices have brought me to a place where each day I can heal. Healing has taught me that pain has purpose. The purpose of our lives is to live with joy.

Joy died when my daughter Emily was killed on the lake in Kelowna. I've gone there every year to celebrate her birthday and honour the day she died. August 8th is a day we celebrate the life she lived. August 26th is the day we mourn and miss her. It's a time to choose to move forward with divine grace. Grace allows us all to heal in our own way, in our own time and to walk together with those we love toward the promise land.

The promise is that we will all heal if we hold steady together. Even when we falter, and when we grieve the loss of the loved we once shared, we can go from lost to found if we stay together and remember the value of family.

I have learned that family can't be bought or bartered with. I know that words hurt, but our hearts heal. I use my words carefully now, and know that I must say what I mean, mean what I say, and never say mean words.

"I love you," is always said before I hang up the phone, walk out the door, or lay my head down to sleep. Each night I pray I will wake to see the rising sun. I rise, I shine, and I look into the mirror with pride, knowing I am living life on my terms. Terms of endearment are what I know must be the foundation upon which I build my life. Family first, family faithful, and the freedom to heal.

"Father and Mother, I Love You," is how I understand family. My father created this world, my mother provides me with everything I need, and I love every reflection of them here on earth. Each precious person given to us is here to teach us lessons. Lessons of pain through the shame, guilt, trauma, tragedy, despair, depression, and anxiety of life, we cannot escape. But each new day and every person we meet can bring hope, inspiration, opportunities, abundance, and grace.

Situations can surface that pull us into the soupy stew of doubt, discouragement, pessimism, fear, and give us a frantic feeling that something is wrong. We are wrong. We can become stuck in a space where we forget why we're suffering.

Other times, suffering is optional. We can try to avoid the pain and choose to paint the canvas of life with what brings us pleasure. Or we can use and abuse every wonderful gift the Great Universal Creator of ONE gives us. We can also blame God for our misfortune. But the truth is, we often fail to use the gifts Mother Nature graced us with. We failed to see the beauty in our life. We complained, we whined, and we did nothing to change our circumstances.

Then the great awakening came, and we were gifted with another chance. One more day to wake up, get up, and create the life we wanted. To see the truth that we are responsible for our own healing.

Some of us chose to heal, while others chose to steal. That will always be the reality until the reality changes. You cannot change what does not want to be changed. You can only change what's necessary if you're willing to use the one common denominator in the equation.

The one common denominator in this life that offers a solution to your problem is you. You can choose to change one part of the puzzle that holds the key to your castle. Admitting that you are unhappy means telling the truth when you have been living a lie.

Be true to your word. If you say you want happiness more than anything else, then act like it. Stop spending your time making money and then making everyone else's life miserable. Stop taking the same path, down the same dusty road, and then complain that you're dirty. Clean up your own act, clean up your own life and clean up your attitude.

Embrace the ugly parts of your life so you can understand what went wrong. If you want to right the wrongs in your life, you must face the ugly truth of what you created. You allowed life to happen to you and now is your opportunity to change.

No one can make you feel fabulous all the time. Life isn't always glorious. You will struggle, but you will survive. Look at how far you've come. Life is filled with an abundance of opportunity and an obstacle course of constant change. You can either choose to drive the car or be a passive passenger. If you don't have a car, you have other options to get to your destination of choice. Pick up your feet and take a leap forward towards the life you want.

Spread your arms, your wings, and your ambitions. Be bold, be brave, be courageous. Above all else, don't be normal.

Recover the part of your life that you have longed to create. Find someone, something, or somewhere that inspires you. Decide what makes you jump for joy and then leap into the belief that creating that is possible. It is possible!

I promise you can become the best possible version of yourself. I guarantee that a life that lights you up is just ahead of you. However, I know the way may be filled with challenges and choosing the correct path may seem difficult. What is illogical, is expecting your life to be happy without taking an active role in creating it, in writing your own story.

My story is written from a place of trauma that could have taken me down a dark path that destroyed me. I took the challenges and wrote a new story. A better story that is filled with love, laughter, and happily ever after. Each day, I wake with a joy that fills my sails, and I am blessed. I would love to take you there too. I would be honored to help you recover your joy!

# CHAPTER 10: Richard Mordern My Journey of Loss and Growth

My journey with Conscious EFT happened by chance in the early spring of 2013. I knew something in my life was not working, but I couldn't put my finger on exactly what I was feeling or why. I just knew that something needed to change.

Learning and exploring new ideas is what I love, so I followed every lead that came into my awareness. I had not yet found anything that resonated until the day I came upon a course given by Nick and Jessica Ortner. The course was an introduction to a modality called EFT.

It felt different, and that intrigued me. I followed the free online course and learned the technique with no awareness of the importance it would play in my life. In the summer of 2013, I lost my wife suddenly. I kissed her goodbye in the morning and on her way to work; she suffered a brain aneurism that left her completely brain dead.

In the space of a few short hours, I went from a happily married man to a single, grieving father of two teenagers. I knew that my role in life had instantly changed. I needed to be present for my children, to help them grieve and move forward into healing. Instinctively, I knew this meant I had to learn to take care of myself first, so that I could be strong and healthy for them.

I turned to EFT. The online course had given me enough knowledge to know that this was a powerful technique. I dug deeper and by October, I had found a 3-day course within driving distance. I immersed myself in learning.

That 3-day course changed me in ways that I am still coming to grips with. I was taught about the role trauma plays in our lives. How it shaped and molded my very existence in ways I couldn't begin to understand. So, I dug deep through the layers of my life.

Trauma can be sudden, like the loss of my wife. Or subtle, like a parent who is overly rigid and firm to the point of abuse. Trauma experiences shape us into the people we are, without really understanding how or why. Over the course of those three days, many life experiences that I had buried rose to the surface. I had to face and ultimately release them yet keep their lessons intact.

I grieved for my wife, my brother who had committed suicide, my father who was unable to show love, and many other situations I had put away in a box labeled life. Until I discovered EFT, I did not realize how powerful these experiences were and how I had adapted my life to suppress them. Emotionally, I had become very pragmatic, resolving myself to take care of the business of life while burying my emotions.

Slowly, I uncovered and healed years of conditioning. After building on that foundation, by the spring of 2014, I began a 10-month course to 'Harness my Power'. I achieved certification as an EFT Practitioner, facilitated by the founder of Conscious EFT, Nancy Forester.

Nancy became and continues to be my mentor. Her guidance and extensive training, gives me a foundation of personal growth and emotional awareness, which has become my strength and my passion in life.

This life-changing sequence of events has changed the course of my life. In 2013, I was still working full time at Honda; my role in quality assurance was a huge disconnect from the awareness and experiences that I was learning about.

I had experienced an uplifting and spiritual change that profoundly changed my outlook on life. Soon enough, my children were heading off to experience higher education and start their lives. My work with them was finished. I'd helped them become the adults that they were destined to be.

I knew I had to let go and allow their lives to unfold and move on with my own path. I opened my heart and realized I now had a calling to help others make a difference in their lives.

The gift of EFT had shaped a new future that allowed me to connect on a much deeper and profound level with those around me. We learn from everyone that comes into our lives, and that is a very important principle we often forget.

After retirement, I wanted to use this knowledge to become more expansive and teach others to live their lives to a fuller extent. My goal then became focused on teaching others how to use the pain that trauma had created in their lives, to become more caring, more compassionate, and to experience more love.

It is not only possible, but it is the foundation of my work. To help others see how essential this is on our journey here. There is no limit to where we can take our lives. I want people to understand they can have everything they long for in life. It takes hard work and the willingness to look beyond the limits of the experience; to see the other side… the awareness, color, sounds, people, and connections.

We can live our life with intention, not giving in to the things that are there to distract us. It is honorable to work with others, but we first need to learn how to work with ourselves. To learn to be aware and loving, despite the trauma. In fact, because of it. Our strength comes from the tragic events that force us to grow.

From our earliest years, ages zero to seven, we form our perceptions of reality on an unconscious level. Every experience is registered in our subconscious and can become a driving force in our life. Each event creates an imprint on us, and these imprints drive our decisions, beliefs, and ultimately our actions.

Often, we are completely unaware that we have even made such a choice. Once the subconscious nervous system makes that decision, it is carried until it is released. The beliefs that make up our story can have a powerful effect on our behaviors. Stories that we unconsciously pick up and tell ourselves can foster patterns of behavior and safeguards that we put into place to avoid feeling negative emotions.

No emotion is truly negative, of course, but our perception that it does not feel nice leads us to protect our emotional self. This protection is simply a trauma; or a painful feeling that was never allowed to run its course and move through our system.

Trauma eventually needs to be processed and negated if we want to be free of the behavior surrounding it. Trauma can happen without awareness and be carried with us for the rest of our lives.

A simple moment of time, like when a child feels unsafe for even an instant, it can cause a lifelong trauma pattern. Imagine a child who has hurt themselves and goes looking for reassurance from their parent. If for any reason—let's say the parents just finished an argument—so the parent is emotionally unavailable. The body of the child may register an emotional reaction to being unsafe. No reassurance was there when it was required.

This event then leaves a mark on the nervous system of the child, and they may unconsciously decide that he is alone and unsafe. Again, this is not a conscious decision, but a fleeting moment that makes a lasting impression.

These nervous system imprints also happen naturally when we face difficult life events that put us in real life danger. Accidents, abuse, ongoing tension from alcohol, drugs, or parental anger issues register in the emotional body as trauma.

PTSD can register any time when a person is faced with deep emotional or long-lasting stressful events. The result is the same. We build those safeguards and patterns of behavior to avoid feeling the pain. These safeguards become our limiting beliefs which directly influence the choice of behavior.

As an EFT Practitioner, I come from a place of compassionate awareness. It is my job to listen to the story, but not become ensconced in it. After much trial and error, I learned the key to working with this energy is to detach from my client's story. We all have a story we tell ourselves to make sense of the world.

I just need to listen to enough of the story to understand and uncover the most important elements. Then I can discover the underlying limiting belief that was created to ease the pain of the trauma.

My overriding concern is that I do not rehash the incident or have the client relive the experience. We don't need to do that to create a new awareness. EFT is not behavioral therapy. It is an interruption of the patterns that have been created.

I help the client uncover a situation where a belief was made via a traumatic memory. Often, the client is totally unaware of the event that created the limiting decision, but the subconscious remembers and responds to them in everyday life events.

A person may not even understand where their unsettled or anxious emotions originate from, but the belief created directly affects their behaviors. In our world, levels of anxiety, stress, and tension are extremely high, and we are unaware of how we are creating and choosing these states of being.

The perceived safety of the client is of utmost concern. Without a feeling of trust, the work cannot proceed. I truly love this work; the process of discovery because it allows me to engage in a much deeper and more compassionate way. I'm more aware of everything around me.

I know I'm not healing your traumas. I'm not healing your PTSD. I am engaging with you in such a way that the transformation is coming from you. I give my client the tools and colors to use, but it's their journey. Think of me as a travel agent; I can suggest multiple routes that will each lead you to the destination that you desire, but that location is your choice.

The healing process takes time. I facilitate the healing, and it is a powerful, humbling position that I am honored to fulfill.

**What is EFT?**

EFT, or the Emotional Freedom Technique, is commonly referred to as "tapping." Essentially, it is a form of psychological acupressure, based on targeting the same points used in traditional acupuncture.

Instead of invasive needles, however, you use your fingertips to tap gently or manipulate the specific meridians of the head and chest while you think about your specific issue. No matter what it may be, while you tap, you recite positive affirmations. This unique combination of tapping and positive affirmations clears the emotional block and restores the harmony between your mind and body. In this way, you can rewire your brain to eliminate the issues caused by the limiting decisions made during times of trauma.

This is a mindless process; in that you do not have to know how it works to get the benefits. When I am teaching EFT to a client, I will start by demonstrating the nine traditional points on the head and upper torso. I also teach them the corresponding finger tapping method.

Simply by tapping on the ends of your fingers, you can calm your system down and drop your cortisol levels. The beauty of finger tapping is that you can literally do it anywhere. Be it driving in the car or conversing with your boss in a tense situation. It is simple, effective, and no one will realize you're performing a self-care activity.

Even without a skilled practitioner, you can use the technique to feel safer, calmer, and more aware as you reduce the overwhelm. Our body is the record holder of our emotions and our stories. As we release the tension from the body, we heal the entire system. A calm system is a healthier system, physically, emotionally, physiology, and neurologically.

I always have my client prepare a record of how they are feeling and what events are going on in their lives that brought them to my office. I often find that as they go through their healing journey, they forget the phobias or behaviors that brought them to me. This can be a powerful tool to highlight the growth and understanding. Many people believe in their own power to heal themselves, because, really, that is the entire point.

I am just a guy who is teaching you a process. You are the one doing the work and creating the lasting changes. I give you the map, but you are the one on the journey.

The next step is to assess their state of mind in regard to the trauma response. Where is the person in the nervous stage? Since everyone reacts differently under stress, I must get an accurate assessment to prepare my client for the work ahead. Each state of mind is approached differently to ensure a positive outcome. For instance, if a client is highly agitated or aggressive, I must first teach them to calm their system down.

Someone who is emotionally frozen in the time of the event would need an entirely different approach than someone who is feeling intense anger. What I don't want is a range of emotions that drag a person all over the map and cause confusion. I need the client to be in a steady, predictable state of mind as we tackle and release them from the limiting belief.

My work is essentially teaching people to be empowered and self-full. In our world, that is considered selfish, but it's not. When you are empowered and have the capacity to care for yourself, you create boundaries. You have awareness, and you can make good choices.

We're so habitual, programmed to take the path of least resistance. We all want to find our comfort zone and hang out there. It may not be the place where we find the most happiness, but it is the place where we understand the limits and have the reassurance that we are safe.

Predictability is safety. We know what to expect and we can find the strength to move through our daily patterns without surprises. Digging into the reasons behind our behaviour is scary, but it is only when we understand why we behave a certain way that we can make a conscious choice for something else. That's more beneficial, and it becomes a choice that you've empowered yourself to make. Even if you felt you didn't have a choice before. I love helping others to open the doors to a new life.

There are a lot of traditional therapies out there. I have known people who have been in therapy for 20-years or more. The traditional idea seems to be that you remove and heal all the pain and trauma before you add in the good stuff. This creates wealthy therapists, but the clients are caught in a never-ending cycle of pain and suffering.

Conscious EFT turns that premise on its head. We teach people how to move forward in a safe, effective manner while preparing the system for the changes ahead. As we work through the process, clients replace the limiting beliefs with a new creation of their own making.

I teach them to consciously chose the future they desire. As they set about creating this future, the old limiting beliefs and patterns fade away until they are unrecognizable. In their place, a new, powerful sense of self emerges.

It's a journey, and it takes time for the client to invest their energy into their lives, sometimes for the very first time. Again, we have been taught it's a very selfish thing to do. But being self-full is the most important thing we can ever do for ourselves.

As we fill up our cup and create a life of happiness and fulfilment, the positive energy spills out to those around us. Each of us feeds the collective with the energy we put out into the world. Let's make that the most loving, healing feeling we possibly can.

The premise of EFT is that we deal with what's happening in our life right now, in the present moment, and work on ways to improve those situations. As we work on the emotional response to a memory, belief, or pattern, you will learn to recognize the story you've been telling yourself. The story that's become such part of you that you have started believing it is you, and all that you can be.

Your story has become your identity and you may not even be aware that it is a creation of your own making. I can teach that you can change the script at any time and create the life you desire. EFT interrupts the emotion behind the story. It redirects the electrical patterns that course though your body, carrying the emotions and reactions to each part of your awareness. You can choose to open the door, release the story with all its attendant emotions and reactions, and move towards something better.

One way, trauma surfaces is through our relationships and communications with our family. Obviously, in every family, we see people in a place of crisis or distress. It may show up as a job loss, an illness, or maybe something serious, like a drug addiction or a child who self-harms.

Our immediate response is to give the most urgent situation all our attention. We can look for a professional to help with the immediate crisis so that our loved one can find some resolution to their immediate pain.

In lots of cases, these family dynamics become a perpetual situation where everyone is coping, and no one is really thriving. Pain becomes the default choice because people do not understand that it is a choice. You can choose pain, or you can choose unhappiness.

You can choose to dwell in an energetic space, never understanding that you have the power to shift your own reality. This is where self-full care enters the picture. We can choose to stay in the same fishbowl, swimming around forever, or we can choose to jump into the ocean.

When one person develops the courage to step out and take care of their own wellness and being, the entire dynamic of the family will change. Emotional wellness starts with you and expands to the rest of the family. That is exactly what happened in my family; my personal journey to wholeness created an environment in which my children could also heal and thrive. As they moved into their new lives, they did so with gratitude and love.

I know I was there for them when they needed me most, and it began by being there for myself first. We have all watched as family members come through a crisis or a depression and appear to return to normal. Everything appears to be fixed, and we heave a sigh of relief and go back to our comfort zone.

The safety measures get put back into place and life goes on much as it did before. But before long, the overwhelm cycle starts again. This is where we need to reset our neurology with a new set of beliefs and habits. To create a new foundation to build from. These new experiences don't just happen, we have to create them.

I have the blueprint of how to get there. You get to supply the details and make it your own incredible journey of life. Those little foundations of success will build upon each other and one day, you will look back in gratitude at everything you have created one step at a time.

As we focus on creating the present, we become stronger, more resilient, and have a greater capacity and awareness. As we near the end of our life journey, we can know that we came at it with the best we had to give. A place of empowerment, safety, and love.

We're human beings, having this wonderful human experience, and we have the gift of free will throughout all of it. It is our choices and experiences that determine who we are. Let us choose to love ourselves first and allow that love to flow freely to everyone we encounter.

In closing, I am not here to say that everything in my life has been rosy and beautiful. Quite the opposite. A lot of powerful, traumatic events led me to where I am today. I've said goodbye to so many people; they all touched my life in different ways, and I hold memories of each of them in a place of awareness and caring.

I understand how experiences that can be perceived as bad, or full of pain, can shape our reality in a myriad of ways. When you let go of the pain and honour the experience, you fill your heart with love.

The memories of a person who has left become richer and full of meaning, giving a shape and depth to life. A year or so after my wife passed, I wrote down a concise description of the next relationship that I intended to create. It was a letting go of the past and a way to honor the love that I had shared with her soul.

I knew what love felt like, and I wanted to experience that again. This time creating something different, but just as powerful. Sure enough, the relationship did manifest, and life evolved into another experience of growth and expansion.

I have become the person I intended to create. You can do that as well; it is not a magic process. When we desire something and do the work of changing our beliefs and our habits, we give over our vibration to something new and greater. EFT is a simple, powerful, and effective tool to make that change.

What do you need to do for you? What's most urgent for you? How many of us are being parents to our parents? Where are you in your life? Work? Play, partners, children, stepchildren, new relationships, new jobs?

Where are the ongoing conflicts or stresses in your life? And, most importantly, what would you like to see different in your life?

I would be happy to have that discussion with you about how to begin to make these changes. It would be my honor.

# CHAPTER 11: Linda Hayes Cooper Rocking the Cradle

***There is no greater agony than bearing an untold story inside you. - Maya Angelou.***

My hope in sharing this chapter is to awaken a curiosity and awareness of early trauma, which we are all exposed to at some level. The power of its impact is not merely determined by its persistence, intensity, and our perception, or more importantly, our disconnect from ourselves and others.

I will give you two examples of perinatal trauma in pregnancy and birth, and share how trauma, along with other conditions, are transgenerationally imprinted on our DNA. The examples provided will for many, be viewed as less significant forms of trauma. Yet they are clear examples of trauma that is formed through disconnect with lasting effects on the individuals' lives.

I want to teach you about the adverse early childhood experiences (ACEs) where a footprint of trauma continues along a path both consciously and subconsciously, throughout our lives. Also, how it affects our physical, emotional, and social-interactive wellbeing across a lifespan, and further if we allow it!

I attended various individual and group sessions on regression hypnosis, ranging from my past life, my own pregnancy, birth, and early childhood experience. Each had a unique, vivid, visual, and somatic effect which seemed to mirror and express as a theme throughout my life.

In these regressions, my experience in the womb and of birthing was vague. A mysterious image of darkness with large deep purple-crimson colours flowed and swirled. At times, it was flat and still.

With guidance, I relaxed deeper, sinking into the couch, my body twitching with periodic involuntary movements. My mind-body struggle subsided as I let go of any expectations, allowing both to come alive in imagery and sensation.

Amongst the swirling shades of black and grey, an image appeared before me, a silhouette of a small baby, sitting in silence in the corner of a cave, looking towards an area of brightness. She was waiting in anticipation for a greeting or movement, yet the silence and stillness surrounded her.

Leaping, like a frog off the soft walls of her enclosure in an attempt to provoke a response, was futile. Suddenly, a shadow generating light, excitement, and warmth filled the space. It was a masculine hand that gently caressed the surrounds of the cave. With this sensation, the tightness and flutter in my chest settled to calm. Yet, as soon as it came into my presence, it faded. Darkness echoed once again within the cave, yet now it transformed into my ribcage, that held a vigorous pounding heart.

I wanted more and more to connect with that warmth again. To see, to hear, and feel its caressing calmness again. A dark image overshadowed the loud pulsing of my aching heart. Overwhelmed with uncertainty, tears of sadness flowed.

My childhood memories are quite rich with feeling and emotion. Happy, easy-going, sun-shining days fill my mind when remembering growing up in the inner suburbs of Sydney in the 1970-80s. Days of playing in the garden, making mud pies, chasing butterflies and kittens, and climbing trees to pick fruit. I cycled the streets with neighbours, built cubby houses with my siblings in the bush, captured cicadas at dusk and stayed up watching them shed their shells. Then, with great excitement, I exchanged the variety of colours with school friends the following day.

Some days, I would hang with Dad stargazing, or join in cleaning the tropical fish tank. I'd watch movies with Mum while she ironed our clothes. On rare occasions, I would enthusiastically delve into a bag of scrap materials looking for surprise pieces for my dolls, whilst Mum sewed dresses for us.

They were 'the good old days.' My father worked and studied, and my mother returned to work once the three of us commenced school. But school was a struggle. My interests were with people and nature rather than academia. What seemed a repeat of the same report card year after year, and my father laying down the rules for study and homework, fell on deaf ears, or should I say, a distracted little girl? However, it didn't seem to bother me, I was happy, easygoing, and I moulded to every situation with ease.

Throughout my midwifery and psychology training, I became curious about my early childhood and gleaned that my parents cared for three young children under 3.5 years with very little support.

I was the middle child and had been born prematurely with milk allergies and intolerances. Soon after my sister was born, my mother was bedbound following a postpartum haemorrhage. Although my parents agreed it was a very busy time, they sheltered me from the finer details of their pain and all the well-known challenges of adjusting to early parenthood.

I knew my mother's father died when she was in junior school and her mother, unable to cope, moved away, leaving her in the care of her grandmother and seven cousins. My mother's relationship with her mother was 'loving' on the surface, but she had little contact in my early years.

In hindsight, I see now how the emotional pain and suffering she endured from their broken bonds, the grief and loss of her mother and father as a young girl, would have been overwhelmingly immense. Especially the inevitable revisiting of these traumas as 'ghost in the nursery', whilst mothering her own 3 young children.

My earliest memories are of her silent presence, not necessarily with me. She moved quietly in the background, providing care for us, yet emotionally unavailable because of her inner sadness and pain.

It was my commencement in prenatal bonding (BA - Bindungs-analyse)* training with Dr. Gerhard Schroth, and Anne Goertz-Schroth over the past year, that allowed an awakening of my pregnancy, birth, and early childhood experiences from my hidden subconscious to a conscious awareness.

This experiential training provided an enriched, detailed memory extending far greater than any conversations I'd had with my parents many years before. The time was right, and I revealed what had never been spoken of. The secret my parents and I shared regarding my birth was kept secret in order to protect me.

This 'trance-formational' work with Gerhard and Anne led me to experience the grief and sadness of being left alone in the womb. Of being birthed early and rapidly alone on a cold surface in darkness. My questioning, "Was I alive?"

Then, I had an image of my tiny body being held up in the cold air toward my mother. Of us both crying and looking at each other. Suddenly, I was whisked away by a stranger and laid out on a trolly. A bright light blinded me. I was watching myself being poked, stabbed, pushed, and pulled as many people watched over. Once again, I felt the pain in my heart of being alone and disconnected.

Captured moments of my early years when I was left alone again, sometimes my cries not answered, curling up alone in my cot weeping myself to sleep. I remembered a comforting memory of my mother reaching down to hold my hand when we were walking down a busy shopping area after preschool. I felt afraid, yet she was there to soothe me in a way that only she knew how to do.

I felt a sense of healing and admiration for Gerhard and Anne being there for me during this process. Offering a safe container in which to open, explore, and heal. Throughout this work, I was able to piece together the puzzle of my early life. The fears, anxieties, struggles, strengths, life experiences, and my love and compassion for my parents.

My mother and I grew very close throughout my adult life, especially following my father's passing. At the time of my regression work, she was suffering from advancing Alzheimer's disease, and I had been grieving her loss through 'anticipatory grief' following her move to senior living.

Given the timing, this regression work was extremely cathartic for me. I was left feeling light, energized, at peace, open, and free, with so much gratitude for my parents.

I received word of my mother's passing from cardiac failure a few days after. What I anticipated my response to be, was far from my actual experience. I accepted my sadness and loss. I left feeling a greater connection, understanding, a deeper love, appreciation, and compassion for my mother and all she had endured. Most of all, I was thankful for her unconditional love, and for accepting me just the way I was, always.

There was unexpected healing and insight for me once I knew the trauma, I experienced from my marriage breakup was like that of my pregnancy and birth experience.

There were many months of disconnect and silence in my marriage as I tried to invoke communication, connection, and intimacy to little effect. Then there was a sudden rupture, cutting of the cord, and removal of what was then my only safe haven.

I was alone, open to the world, cold, shaken, and wounded. I endured many days of suffering, vulnerability, and being alone with medical and psychological interventions.

What was also fascinating, and possibly brought about my sense of freedom and peace, was the subsiding of my subconscious, involuntary ideomotor movements. My body jerked and quivered when in a deep, relaxed, meditative, or trance-like state. This bodily response began after the traumatic experience of my marriage break up six years ago.

I experienced those involuntary movements intensely whilst in training over my week with Gerhard and Anna. I have not experienced them since. Peter Levine (2017) speaks of these involuntary movements as the body's way of regulating itself to bring it back to balance. The state which can occur through reassuring social engagement of safety.

It was Gerhard and Anne's safe container with offerings of their gentle, caring, and safe presence that allowed this process to occur. My body cleaned out and healed any remaining trauma wounds from these life experiences.

Early imprinting and attachment studies date back to Lorenz (1935) and Bowlby (1969). Decades of evidence have followed since, pressing the awareness of healthy early infant development, and bonding to prevent long-term physical, social, and emotional harm.

A mother's emotional state shapes the baby's brain, whether it is fear, sadness, happiness, love, or anger. The stress we express when we have challenges can be resourceful, yet if intense, with persistent pressure, can be too much for the developing brain to manage.

In the womb, infants take on board the stress on a cellular level through their senses. A sense of self and temperament can be influenced and can be temporarily wired in. Bruce Lipton's work on cellular memory supports epigenetics—meaning the DNA does not change, only the expression of it changes. He mentions two types of DNA, the chromosomal DNA that makes up 2% and determines eye colour, skin, stature, etc.

The second is noncoding DNA responsible for behaviour, emotions, and personality traits that we inherit. The noncoding DNA is affected by stressors in the environment, such as emotions, toxins, and inadequate essentials like nutrition. Some of the epigenetic information is downloaded in the cells of the sperm and egg that have a potential to be passed on and expressed.

Dr. Brian Weiss speaks of a young boy whose family enlisted his help for their young son who was self-harming by hitting his head against objects. The family history enlightened them to his grandfather's capture and torture, repetitive beatings about the head by the Khmer Rouge (communist party of Kampuchea).

Following disclosure and discussion of this with their son, the self-harming behaviour ceased. In many ways, epigenetic changes are tools that prepare us for the stressors and the traumas our parents experienced. For good, they play down the traumatic experiences of our biological family history, but on the other hand, the express it. Rachel Yehuda calls these intrinsic tools our 'environmental resilience', as they are a means of preparing us to adapt for survival.

As its existence, it lives on a cellular level either through non-coding DNA, or current environmental circumstances. Its wound shows the scar on an emotional, psychological, and physiological level. Deep within, it affects our neurobiology, our nervous system, and our immune system, setting up for unhealthy disease states and conditions that may be expressed at any time over the lifespan.

If the levels of stress are high, the most common are PTSD, mental illness, personality disorders, addictions, cardiac disease, ADHD/ADD, auto-immune diseases, asthma, diabetes type 1, cancer, chronic pain, arthritis (The CDC 1995-1997).

To manage a stressful environment and survive, babies adopt early strategies which they employ to stay connected with their carers to ensure their needs are met. We know these as physical characteristics like large eyes, cute round faces, and crying. Yet they can also behave with subtle reactions and behaviours.

Take, for example, ADD/ADHD. It is thought this condition develops when a mother's deficit of attention to her infant—from conception to 3-years—is persistent enough that disconnect is traumatic for the infant. The infant may develop a strategy of tuning out, or attempting engagement through hyperactive activity, resulting in ADD and ADHD patterns, respectively.

Gabor Mate in his book *Scattered Minds* (2018) speaks of this adaptation. From an attachment viewpoint, the grandparents of attachment—John Bowlby and Mary Ainsworth—along with one of their research colleagues, Patricia Crittenden (now DMM attachment and adaptation), studied parent-infant dyads.

They found that infants adapted strategies in relationship with their caregivers' patterns for safety and survival. So, a baby may learn to display only positive emotions around his mother to keep their connection, if she reacts insensitively to his crying or thrashing behaviour.

As we develop levels of sensitivity and awareness to our environment, adopt tools for our survival and adaptation, we form the characteristics of our personality. How they form depends on what our relationships are like with others.

A characteristic that may be seen as imperfect or negative to one person is a strength to another. For example, people with ADHD/ADD are often perceived as lazy with lower intelligence, just because they work and behave differently to others. They are highly intelligent and creative individuals, more so than their non-ADD/ADHD peers. They may take longer due to greater distractibility, yet usually end up having more tasks attended to as they tend to take on more.

Some successful people who were unable to function in school and academic environments due to their ADD/ADHD condition include Leonardo Da Vinci, Albert Einstein, Richard Branson, Bill Gates, and Walt Disney.

In 2016, over 6.1 million children in the USA alone had been diagnosed with ADD/ADHD. The numbers, however, had dropped from 6.4 million in 2011 (Center for Disease Control/CDC, USA).

What is most important for children experiencing ADD/ADHD symptoms is to have an attuned, sensitively responsive parent or carers who see their strengths and weaknesses. They need to feel accepted, encouraged, and supported in their everyday experiences. In my experience, many parents present with questions and concerns regarding the preschooler who is 'different and challenging', being less attentive or hyperactive.

In the following years, they may seek a diagnosis and/or medication for ADD/ADHD. However, providing attention externally for what they lack within is key. Such as using focused tasks and techniques, mindfulness practices, sports, and creative outlets. These will assist them, and encourage them to flourish, rather than them falling victim. In my opinion, ADD/ADHD is a label that is often not helpful to a young person's sense of self, identity, or capacity to flourish.

Adverse Childhood Experiences (ACEs) are situations and events where children from pregnancy through to 17-years are exposed to traumatic events. These can be emotional and physical violence, abuse, or neglect. This includes witnessing (seeing or hearing) distressing arguments or separation, violence, attempted suicide, incarceration, and death.

Another aspect of great impact that is often ignored or played down, are situations that undermine and disrespect the child's sense of self. Their bonding and belonging, safety, and stability. In the heart of all these factors, again, is the disconnect in the relationship.

The Center for Disease Control (CDC) conducts ACE studies, with the initial study reported in 1995-1997. Their survey reported 61% of adults across 25 U.S. states to be experiencing at least one type of ACE, and close to 1 in 6 reported experiencing four or more types of ACEs. Children born to women experiencing four or more types of ACEs were at greater risk of exposure to ACEs.

The CDC (1995-1997) reported households experiencing greater levels of stress, instability, substance abuse, and mental health problems, to have more occurrences of ACEs. In these households, understandably, the focus on the child's need for a loving connection is minimized.

In his book *The Body Keeps the Score* (2014), Bessel van der Kolk reported that victims who witnessed and experienced 9/11 at ground zero and who had loving, sensitive caring relationships around them offering support did not develop PTSD. As opposed to their counterparts with limited emotional and social supports. Interestingly, couples where one or both partners had PTSD tended to experience greater anger, severe conflict, and increased cardiovascular reactions than couples without PTSD (CDC, 1995-1997).

You can find out more about the ACE's study, causes, trajectory, and prevention in the reference link[19]

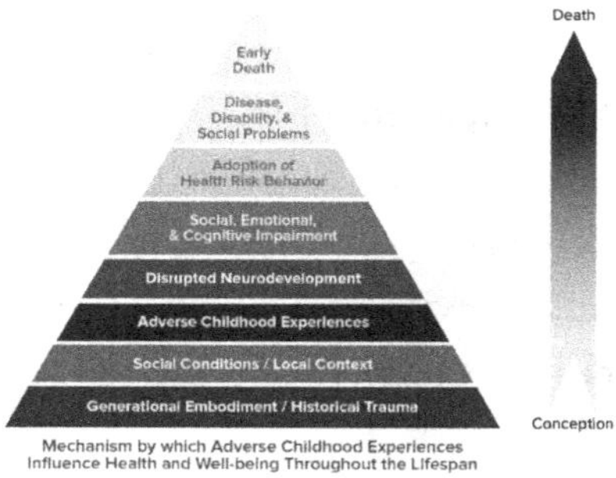
Death
Early
Death
Disease,
Disability, &
Social Problems
Adoption of
Health Risk Behavior
Social, Emotional,
& Cognitive Impairment
Disrupted Neurodevelopment
Adverse Childhood Experiences
Social Conditions / Local Context
Generational Embodiment / Historical Trauma
Conception
Mechanism by which Adverse Childhood Experiences
Influence Health and Well-being Throughout the Lifespan

Diagram 1. The mechanism of ACEs influencing health & well-being across the lifespan.

**Case Study: PTSD - When Trauma Lives on in the Eye of the Beholder.**

Julie was softly spoken, warm, polite, and gentle natured. She was dressed fashionably in a bright summer dress, her makeup and hair perfectly groomed, with long blonde locks flowing over her shoulders. Her polite, cheerful nature was contagious. As we talked, I noticed every response to a question was skewed positively. Her facial expression and intonation of voice was "over-bright and cheery."

There was no hint of negativity voiced on her part or toward any other person. No anger, fear, frustration, blame, guilt, or even sadness. She remained positive in all manner of expressions, until she looked away from my gaze. There it was. Her pain. I got a brief glimpse of her internal world that was released and manifested on her face without her conscious awareness. She wiped her tears with her crumpled tissue as we sat together in silence.

After inhaling a deep breath, she described the events of Sunday evening 4 weeks ago. She was looking after her friend's son. Her son and friend were playing in the garden when she heard a heart-wrenching scream. The kind that no mother wants to hear. She knew immediately it wasn't her son; it was Kye.

He'd fallen on the concrete and split his forehead open. She didn't know what to do. She couldn't get in contact with the mother since the mother was busy at work. So, she comforted him, placed a cloth over his head and got some ice. Then she packed the two children in the car, and just started driving to the hospital.

As she was driving, she suddenly felt woozy. Her heart pounded in her chest, and she knew she was spiralling into a panic attack. Her face was taut as she struggled to hold back the tears while she described the tension, she'd felt in her hands from squeezing the steering wheel so tight.

In the room with me, her body was mimicking these experiences while she described them. She informed me, she had avoided that route for 5-years because it led to the hospital where Joshua (her son) was born.

"I never go there because it's too painful," she said. "There's too many bad memories." Julie had been referred by her obstetrician-gynaecologist for help with her anxiety and worry.

Steve, her husband, was concerned about her ever-increasing anxious behaviour, difficulty sleeping, irritability, and a general disconnect from her usual self and activities. "Her mind is elsewhere," he reported.

Julie knew she wasn't herself. She even had difficulty watching "The Midwife" documentary on pregnancy and birthing, or hearing others talk about their birth experiences. Frozen in place, she felt her heart pounding in her chest, restricting her to shallow breathing.

She found herself changing the channel briefly, or if her husband was watching, she'd remove herself from the room and distract herself with cleaning to help settle her nerves. Julie reported still having re-occurring, vivid dreams of her labour, just as she had experienced on and off ever since Joshua's birth.

She was pleased to know Joshua cared for her by the statements he made.

"It's okay, Mummy," and "Don't worry, Mummy," he said as he gave her extra hugs, food, and pictures he had drawn for her. However, it kept happening frequently. It wasn't good for him to be put into a position where he needed to look after her.

From her history, I ascertained that her early childhood was fairly common. There were no significant traumatic events. However, I noted her relationship with her mother. She reported situations where she had to please her mother by being happy, polite, and in a constant state of positivity. Otherwise, her mother would get angry, become silent, and avoid her. Julie disliked anything negative, especially any confronting situations. She never complained or showed negative emotions, such as sadness, anger, yelling, or frustration around her mother.

She skimmed over her labour, and birth experience like it was a series of procedural events.

"They never offered me pain relief," she said. "They just kept saying how great I was doing. I was in so much pain." Yet, it seemed like she never asked for any.

It was as though the midwives were supporting her through it. Yet from Julie's view nothing could be further from the truth. My thoughts entertained the view that even in labour, she was still wearing her happy mask. Her learnt behaviour of staying connected to carers, to not display any negative view or emotions, to please and be the good girl, had then played out in the relationship between her and the maternity staff.

Julie had experienced PTSD, or PTI (Post Traumatic Injury, as Peter Levine describes) since Joshua's birth 5-years earlier. Julie's inability to connect and share her concerns and need for pain relief during labour, led to a relational disconnect at a time when she needed connection most.

Her heightened stress, pain, and fear activated her nervous system to release the fight, flight, freeze, or faint responses. Her body's surges of cortisol and adrenaline hormones brought on a fear of death. Over the years, she had calmed her nerves with medication and avoidance. It was merely a Band-Aid that had been ripped off when she needed to return to the same hospital setting where her initial trauma was downloaded into her system.

Julie and I worked on her healing in various ways. However, first she needed to be heard, to be seen, and validated. She needed to know I was connected and would be there for her. When people speak of their adversities and trauma, they speak factually rather than emotionally, left brain versus right brain. This is where we began. (You can access a PDF describing this process via emailing me through my website)[20].

MiCBT - Mindfulness meditation is a body-focused right brain approach for reprogramming her anxiety and depression. This includes imagery exposure, somatic bodywork, and Interoceptive signature, which allows the experience of sitting with the negative emotions and sensations as they rise. The object is to accept the fall and dissipation mindfully until reaching a window of calm and equilibrium.

Julie worked with me for 6-months and continued her growth throughout the year. She contacted me at the end of the year with news that she was pregnant and excited to follow our plan for her birth experience. She would have a supportive team who were in the know about her experience. They would provide the resources she requested and help her towards a better outcome.

In summary, trauma is all around. It lurks, not unlike the unknown within the ocean. Once we are in it, we test the waters; we take a dip, dive, swim, and splash around playfully. At times, we pause to ease our way in, maybe catch our breath, or we are thrown into the deep end.

How we mange the impact of the ocean is determined by our ability to draw on our resources, resilience, and support of others to help us ride the wave. When the swell rises, the lifeguard throws that lifeline of connection to you and brings you to safety and calm. *Prenatal Bonding (BA), Gerhard and Anne Schroth Germany. Its origins are from a Hungarian psychoanalyst, Dr. Jenoe Raffi, early 1990's.

# CHAPTER 12: Roseline Salazar Recovery: Journey After the Military

When military service members are deployed or at war, they are exposed to potentially traumatic events. Some of these include life-threatening combat situations, witnessing injury or death, killing, or wounding the enemy, being involved in serious motor vehicle accidents, or even handling human remains.

Research has proven a strong link between levels of combat stress and PTSD. Their minds are conditioned to be on alert around the clock. In addition, other factors can increase their chances of developing PTSD or other mental health problems. Another cause of stress is military sexual trauma (MST). This is sexual assault or repeated, threatening sexual harassment that occurs in the military. It can happen to men and women. MST can occur during peacetime, training, or war.

I underwent ten weeks of strenuous combat skills training (CST). It included, but wasn't limited to, formations, physical fitness, weapons, High Mobility Multipurpose Wheeled Vehicle (HMNWV) rollover, carrying rucksacks, and more. We were training for war.

At the end of my training, I was deployed to Camp Clark, Khowst, Afghanistan, from December 2008–December 2009. It took approximately two weeks before we finally arrived at our so-called home. I realized then, my fellow military brothers and sisters would be my family for the upcoming year.

Meeting the group and getting to know them was a little uncomfortable because most of the group were Army soldiers, with only a few Navy personnel, and Air Force airmen like myself. There were about eight females, and the rest were all men. Total numbers at Camp Clark were approximately 200, which included mechanic and food service contractors.

About four days after arriving, I went on my first supply run. We traveled with four vehicles with at least 12 personnel, or 6 MRAPS, with at least eighteen personnel.

I was the driver of the S4 MRAP, which just means the vehicle for our camp. A normal supply run involved bringing back equipment parts, such as MRAP and HMMWV tires and spare parts on our 5-ton truck. We also picked up mail from families that were to be passed out at our camp.

Going on my first supply run was great because I was excited to see what it looked like outside of camp. I was curious to see what kinds of homes were there, and what the families looked like. I finally saw a group of sheeps, goats and other farm animals following their leader.

When we first arrived, the rules dictated that each convoy had to have at least six vehicles, with at least three personnel per vehicle when going on supply runs or battlefield circulations.

A battlefield circulation happened when our camp chief had meetings with the elders and other leaders. Orders came that required us to travel to their location. During the night hours, anywhere between 7 p.m. and 5 a.m., we had incoming attacks, whether it was rockets or mortars.

Almost every day we got attacked during the night hours anywhere from twice to five times. It was hard to have a decent sleep because we never knew when the Taliban would strike next or if one of us would be killed. Sleep was imperative as we still went on convoys four to six times a week. Unfortunately, this was part of what we signed up for and we just had to do our best.

In addition to the stress of being attacked, going on convoys, and not knowing if we would live another day, I experienced what others in my camp didn't. Workplace bullying.

Something weird happened when I arrived at our camp. I needed to use the latrine (restroom), and as I walked into the dining facility, this gentleman was walking out. I had a bad feeling about him; I sensed trouble.

When I asked him where the restrooms were located, he responded politely while pointing in the direction I needed to go. I went to the restroom and decided I would call it a night.

The next morning, I reported to my work section bright and early and learned that the gentlemen I'd spoken with, was going to be my boss for the rest of the year. It was an eerie feeling, but I told myself to give him the benefit of the doubt. I had no choice but to work with him.

There were many times when we headed through downtown Khowst to our destination. I will not forget one run we went on; I was the truck commander (TC) of our 5-ton vehicle. The TC is the person who listens in and responds to the convoy commander through our radios.

The roads were crowded that day, so once we reached town, and saw the amount of people blocking our way, we slowed down. There were no locks on the doors of our 5-ton, so we ended up holding onto them as tight as we could. The driver held his steering wheel and his door.

Our gunner struggled with the turret because it wasn't easy to turn. While making our way through, we realized we were being ambushed. With people everywhere, I couldn't distinguish between who was innocent and who was the enemy. Since I never experienced an ambush before, I can honestly say this was, and still is, the scariest experience I've had, and I am forever damaged by it.

What should have been an 8-hour convoy ended up being six-hours of ambush and another five long hours to get back to our camp. I thank God we got back to our camps safe and sound. As tired as I was, I couldn't sleep. I felt traumatized. But like everyone else, we had to continue and head out on more convoys.

There were a few deaths at our camp during my deployment, which still and will forever affect me. Around a month after I arrived at my camp, the group before me was getting ready to start their journey back home to the United States.

Two weeks before their final departure, they were transporting equipment to a forward operating base, where they would make their flight to Kabul. The convoy was destroyed by a vehicle-borne improvised explosive device (VBIED). Two members died, one was paralyzed from the waist down, and one was burnt to death. The TC hit the roof of the HMWV, the gunner flew off with the turret landing on him and he died instantly.

After receiving the news, I realized how much danger our lives were in. Four more lost their lives during my time at Camp Clark, which were very traumatizing. But this is what I signed up for, so I just had no choice but to keep my faith and stay strong.

After the death of our first sergeant that occurred midway into my one-year deployment, I started my first therapy session. I was escorted to a nearby camp where medical attention was available. I didn't trust my first therapist because he was a male, and I needed counsel for combat trauma and being bullied by males. But after my third session, I felt more at ease.

I felt like he believed me about the bullying and showed sympathy for my traumatic experience. It was then I knew treatment was necessary and not a joke like I thought it was prior to my deployment. After this experience, I promote therapy for the mental health.

Halfway through my therapy, I learned I was relocating to Forward Operating Base (FOB) Lighting in Gardez City. It was nice to see new faces and have a different work pace. I thought I was free from worrying about my new boss, but I was wrong. I was surrounded by members who went to CST with my former boss. The one who bullied me.

Regardless of who was there, I filed a harassment case against him. A medical officer was assigned to my case, and he left to interview personnel at Camp Clark. There were about thirteen witnesses. Three denied any wrongdoings, although they knew exactly what was going on. Some didn't want to be interviewed at all, and this was where I felt even more betrayed.

After a long crucial four-months of waiting, we finally got the verdict. As I've said previously, my case was invalid because I wasn't assigned a lawyer to lead the investigation.

I lost it! I was hurt, angry, and I wanted revenge. All my former boss got was a general letter of reprimand, which is just a slap on the wrist. But I decided I wasn't going to give up. This verdict also motivated me to stand up for women who've been through similar situations. I knew I had a mission to accomplish once I got back to the U.S. That came with a mix of emotions, but despite all that happened, I was just happy to be leaving Afghanistan and going home.

Once we were back on U.S. soil, I signed into my squadron and left to go to my new duty station in my hometown, Honolulu, HI. I learned strategies and techniques to help me cope with the challenging times of my recovery. I was so glad I was going to be stationed with family and have a fresh, new start.

Upon my arrival at my new duty station, I continued treatment. I met my new therapist, who played a huge role in my life. Like meeting a new doctor, we went through the regular intake and turnover. I immediately knew that she'd be a wonderful person to work with.

My therapist continued working with me until I accepted the past and realized, I had no choice but to start the healing process and move on. She helped me prepare for the new life ahead of me, becoming a civilian. When they told me that news, it wasn't great. But it was going to happen whether I wanted it to or not. It was just another step in my healing journey.

**My Post-Traumatic Stress Disorder (PTSD) Diagnosis**

About three months into my treatment, I was diagnosed with PTSD. I was speechless and horrified because I had some idea where it was leading me: to medical discharge. It was very disappointing, considering I worked so hard all those years with plans to retire. But because of my deployment to Afghanistan, my dream career was cut short.

Prior to my deployment, I was fun and outgoing. I loved to attend gatherings and go to the movies. I was enthusiastic about having fun, like normal people do. When I first heard of PTSD during my deployment, I thought it was some prank because others in my camp would joke about it. When I was diagnosed with it, I learned how different I had become due to my combat and harassment trauma.

These were my typical PTSD symptoms:

- Isolating myself (also known as detachment).
- Being on edge and getting easily upset.
- Experiencing nightmares, flashbacks, and reliving the past when triggered.
- No longer interested in activities I used to do.
- Trouble sleeping or insomnia.
- Being startled easily.
- Zoning out or poor concentration.
- Being constantly on guard.
- Getting upset when something reminds me of my experiences.
- Avoiding certain places, people, and things that trigger flashbacks.
- Experiencing suicidal thoughts.
- Depression.

To start my healing journey, I had to accept that I had PTSD, be willing to face the treatment knowing it would be difficult, and stop being afraid of the unknown. Another scary feeling was not knowing what my future would be.

Question after question kept popping into my mind: What would I do after I got out? What would my life be like? The fear grew. The military was my identity, and it was about to be stripped away from me.

During therapy, I also learned the importance of breathing techniques and practicing mindfulness. I made mindfulness a priority by committing to 3-5 five minutes of mindfulness for 30-days. I started my daily mindfulness practice by making a to-do list to ensure positive results.

My to-do list consisted of:

- Creating a comfortable sacred space to meditate in.
- Exchanging my bad habits for good ones.
- Picking a buddy to partner with and then holding each other accountable.
- Letting go of expectations and lifting my limits.
- Being kind to myself

This was just the beginning, but I put my trust in God and depended on my therapist to help me through.

## Upward Spiral Through Therapy

I started my treatment plan and had both good and bad days. But when days were bad, they were terrible. One of the three types of therapy I used was Exposure Therapy. Whenever I had to face a difficult situation, I had either a fight (stay and deal with it) or flight (run away and avoid) reaction.

There were a few times when I got defensive as well. My therapist told me to do whatever I needed to do, but I acted hard-headed like it didn't bother me. This led to a fight with my therapist.

Other times, I felt like running out because the subject was so painful. But I had nowhere to go, so I would just sit there and cry, not saying a word. No matter how my sessions were, I did not give up. I faced some difficult obstacles, and I had setbacks. Two of my biggest were fear and avoidance.

My mind would play tricks on me. I wouldn't do the assignments as instructed, resulting in avoiding the whole situation. One example was getting psyched up to grocery shopping. But the fear of crowds and parked cars caused me anxiety, so I didn't go and failed my assignment.

I also experienced setbacks, such as going backward because of a flashback or a trigger. After our deployment, I feared driving in traffic, seeing certain types of vehicles, or even objects on the side of the road because they reminded me of my combat experiences.

One day, while driving home from work, I saw an empty soda can on the side of the road. I freaked out and pulled over at the next parking lot because it reminded me of a soda can bomb that went off on one of our supply runs.

After this, I stopped driving for a month until I felt comfortable again. I practiced mindfulness and slowly got back on track. I knew obstacles and setbacks were normal, as our healing journey is often described as a rollercoaster ride. But I was determined. Even though I felt like I lost a battle, I kept a positive attitude and kept moving forward.

### The Power of Prayer

Enduring several painful experiences helped me realize my strength and worth. I doubted myself at times and felt as if I was being punished. I couldn't help but wonder why God would put me through such horrible experiences. I wondered if He would help me through. I was angry and lost my faith in Him.

During my deployment, I was told that I ended up at Camp Clark because I was being punished. I thought only an evil person would say that. But over time, a lot of negative events happened one after the other, so I couldn't help but think it was true.

My mental and physical health declined. I hated life and wished I could hit a rewind button, even though, in reality, I knew that wasn't possible. I had a roommate who was aware of my ongoing issues and told me to pray.

One night, she sat me down and explained the reasons I needed to talk to God. She also mentioned that we were all in the same boat and turning to each other for strength was what we were told to do.

She reminded me that God is our creator and redeemer. I realized she was talking to me through God. She held my hand, and we prayed. I then felt a tremendous sense of relief and could now hold my head up high. I was ready to face another day knowing that God was always with me, guiding me through people like my roommate.

I faced a lot of trying times while in the military, especially when my faith was tested just trying to survive. After this experience, I believed we are all on the right track to healing and happiness if we continue to pray.

These were two verses I referred to during challenging times:

***"Ask, and it shall be given to you; seek, and ye shall find; knock, and it shall be opened for you." Matthew 7:7.***

***"With God all things are possible." Matthew 19:26.***

**Path to a Successful Transition**

There were times when I was at my lowest point and almost gave up. I felt as if the world was against me. Being away from family too was tough, but I applied what I was taught as a child. Do your best and never give up. I gained knowledge and life experience while away.

No matter what your career field, or where you are in your healing journey, or what the circumstances are, stay on track with the healing process and stick to your goals. By now, you should already know what you need to do, how to do it, and be able to apply everything it takes to achieve success. Today, you are one step closer to reaching your goal towards having a wonderful life.

During your toughest times, I recommend you keep an open mind and consider mental health treatment as one of your options. Once you start therapy, it's also important to follow through with your treatment plan and not give up. Missing just one session can cause a delay and lead to negative results.

After starting therapy, I made a promise to myself that I would stick to progression and not regression. That wasn't always easy, and I had a few setbacks. Life after the military was very challenging, but I reminded myself the only way to get ahead is to keep going. Stay positive and see every day as a blessing.

**Recovery, Rebuilding, and Persevering**

The road to recovery is a big step–it allows you to leave the past behind and move on to your next chapter in life. I was determined to overcome these obstacles and refused to let the past ruin future opportunities that would lead me to happiness and success.

I had my mind set to build a foundation and rebuild my life in order to set an example for my kids and reach my long-term goals. I now have tools, strength, courage, and support, so nothing holds me back.

I set the bar high and will do whatever it takes to reach it. My experiences made me who I am today, and no one can take that away from me. Nor can they knock me down. There will be obstacles, but there is nothing I can't handle. I went through too much to let anyone rob me of my success and happiness now.

Keep on striving to be the best you can be. When you fall, the only way forward is to pick yourself up. Gather all your anger, frustrations, negative emotions, and pain to boost yourself up. Today, I feel confident. I'm back to doing things that used to make me happy. When challenges come, I overcome them. I feel proud that I've come so far.

I know that no matter what happens in my life now, learning to persevere will help me achieve my goal of transitioning smoothly into civilian life.

# CHAPTER 13: Maricelly Ramos Survive to Thrive

From the age of 15, I was in multiple abusive relationships. After many years of traumatic events, I developed symptoms of PTSD. There were times I couldn't function because of fear, anxiety, and triggers. They took over.

If anyone walked behind me or yelled at me, I would be so afraid that they'd grab me. If I saw anyone who looked like one of my abusers, I got so scared, and my heart would play up. Even if someone looked me straight in the eyes, fear took hold.

One of my abusers used his scary, yellow, and red deep eyes to scare me. Someone told me once that when you tell yourself things, you start to believe them. So, I changed the narrative.

"He's not around," I said. "You are safe, he's no longer going to hurt you."

I wasn't really a person to show too much affection. I didn't want anyone touching me because I was too scared, they 'd hurt me. When people got too close to me, even if it was just to have a simple conversation, I would shake from fear. When I had these triggers, my anxiety was uncontrollable.

One of the first things I learned was to identify my triggers. Even after I learned what they were, I still didn't know how to manage or control them. I lived in constant fear of something happening to me. I was too afraid to start a relationship with anyone because I thought they are going to hurt me. My PTSD was constant, and controlled every area of my daily life, and that wasn't how I wanted to live my life.

This is normal for someone who's been through these types of traumas. I didn't feel peaceful, even in my own home. I lived with constant fear, even though it was just me and the kids living there. My PTSD didn't understand it was my safe space.

I constantly looked behind me, even if it was my children who stood behind me, I didn't feel safe. I was always afraid, unhappy and my anxiety was always on the rise. My chest was consistently tight from the fear of seeing things that weren't there.

I had a choice to make. I could choose to allow the PTSD to control me, or I control it. So, I decided to not let fear define me any longer. I sat down one evening with my affirmation journal and began Expressive Writing. I wrote a list of everything that made me scared, and how I felt during those times of fear.

Then I could identify each trigger and take a step forward into controlling them, instead of letting them control me. The more I wrote things down, the more powerful I felt. Why? Because I chose to no longer let PTSD ruin my life. I still have triggers, but now I am aware of them and understand them. I know what to do when they arise.

I read a lot of self-help books and learned Square Breathing. That's when you breathe in for 4-seconds slowly, hold your breath for 4-seconds, breathe out for 4-seconds slowly, and hold your breath for 4-seconds. To concentrate, I close my eyes and concentrate on my breathing.

It took time, but eventually I got through the difficult times because of it, and a few other coping skills. If you suffer from PTSD, it's important that you identify your triggers and learn to control them, so they don't control you.

I still use Expressive Writing, especially when I feel anxious or triggered. I go for a walk and read self-help books. Listening to music relaxes my mind and helps me get my feelings and emotions together.

The more I learn about this condition, the more I can apply to my daily routine.

That daily routine is the one thing that has worked for me. I've made it a habit to read my affirmations, make my bed, take a warm bath, and go for a morning walk to get my thoughts together before I start my day. Each day, I also journal my triggers and the situation, place, or person who provoked them.

At night, I also take a warm bath or shower, light some Mind & Body candles, and turn my diffuser on with relaxing oils. Lavender is one of my favorites. Then I set up my bed area in a way that helps me to relax.

If you want to heal from your traumas, it starts by wanting to change things within you. To find what triggers you and really commit to learning how to manage them. Many times, we are afraid to confront our nightmares or our fears. But remember, you might not get closure from it, or even need closure. You may just need to give yourself permission to move on, to start over, and to find that peace within yourself and your surroundings.

After many years of suffering from anxiety and having PTSD disturb my daily living, I decided to find my power and get it back. I found inner peace and created peace around me. Yes, it took me years to find it, but when you really want change, you do your best to find out what you need and execute that change.

Don't be afraid to fight your battles, or they will fight you and win. I had to walk away from fear and learn to control my emotions. Now they don't affect me in the same way. It takes discipline to achieve mental health and accomplishing goals to achieve healing. Identify your fears and triggers, then work on each one individually at your pace. Don't rush.

The healing process can be challenging. Sometimes we can get so angry about all the abuse or the traumatic events we've suffered, that we refuse healing and change altogether. We can feel as if we have betrayed ourselves because we chose to forgive, let go, and heal. But forgiving others is for your sake. It's not about them.

The best thing you can do is choose to let go of your past pain. This brings the freedom you need to build a new future. Then forgive yourself for allowing others to hurt you. Be kind to yourself and know it is not your fault.

When I was writing my book *Who Was She?* I realised how much anger I was holding in my heart, and how many tears I'd been holding onto for years. It was hard going back and forth with my past, but so rewarding. I was able to figure out so many things about myself and others and was able to dig deep and find my triggers.

It feels so amazing to have the opportunity to rebirth my life again. To learn how to love myself, accept the past, and build a bright new future. One thing I've learned on this healing journey is how very important it is to let go and live. I encourage you to seek mental help when it's needed. I did, and it was the reason I've been able to heal.

We can't be afraid to find healing within and start over. Remember, you are doing this for yourself, because you deserve a life full of joy and less worry. When you find the strength to let go and allow yourself to pursue healing, you are giving yourself and your children the best gift you can ever give.

Many of the symptoms of PTSD can be different for everyone. I experienced anxiety, flashbacks, guilt, hostility, social isolation, nightmares, insomnia, and unwanted thoughts. I encourage you to try Expressive Writing. It can help you to learn process your feelings.

When I decided to write my memoir *Who Is She?* it was difficult because I had to rewrite the sorrow of my life all over again. It reopened those scars, but also it gave me a chance to get to know who I am and my worth. I was able to heal all my wounds, manage my triggers, and start over.

You can overcome many adversities if you really give yourself a chance to let go, learn, and grow. Many of us who experience a traumatic event or multiple events are terrified of confronting our fears. We are afraid to even think about certain moments that changed our lives forever. I always say either you confront your fears and triggers, or they will confront you and make your life miserable.

I know it can be extremely difficult to think back to the events that caused us so much pain. I have been there. But at some point, in our lives, we have to be held accountable for allowing ourselves to accept less than we deserve.

PTSD triggers are like a ticking bomb. You don't know when it is going to go off, and it can destroy you. It is very important to surround yourself with positive people, to cut off anything that reminds you of your past that is hindering your journey to becoming a better person.

You want to build a new life; you could try joining a support group that is based on similar emotional struggles. Trust yourself that you can overcome anything. Practice positivity and avoid anything that is negative. Then you will find your peace.

I love nature. I enjoy the peaceful environment that helps me concentrate on my breathing. It's beneficial to relax in moments when I'm triggered. Physical activity is important because it helps draw out negative energy, fear, and suffering.

When you leave your trauma and PTSD untreated, it's very unlikely to disappear. It can contribute to a life full of depression, sleep problems, negatively interacting with others, and inhibit the ability to enjoy the life you deserve.

Around 7.7 million adults in the U.S. live with PTSD[21]. Women are twice as likely as men to develop this condition. PTSD can last for many years, and its symptoms can affect your quality of life.

I made sure my social support system is always positive. That there's a good vibe and people who have good energy. Get rid of anything or anyone who doesn't support you or bring positivity into your life.

I practice meditation a few times a week to help me relax. It gets my mind and thoughts off anything that's hurting me or stressing me out. I find a quiet space at home, light some candles, and play positive music. I close my eyes and imagine I am somewhere wonderful. Sometimes it's a place I've never been to before. I let my mind go on vacation.

There are certain scents that can also help ease your mind from your triggers. I use lavender, eucalyptus, rose, sweet orange, sandalwood, and sage in my aromatherapy diffuser. Find a few friends to go to art classes and paint. Art helps you focus and relax, just like meditation. Find what makes you happy. A place at home or a place somewhere you can relax and be yourself. Then breathe in the fresh air and enjoy the sun.

Open your windows and your curtains and enjoy the sun. Reconnect with yourself as many times as needed. Learn ways to manage yourself.

It's understandable that at times, we want to hide our emotional issues and pretend things are normal. Even when deep inside, we are struggling and screaming for help. But we have to heal our inner selves if we want to have a pure soul and be ready for new beginnings.

Every day, tell yourself that you've got this. That you're capable of healing, capable of rebirthing your life again. Do what it takes to change. Others hurt us, but we are responsible for healing ourselves. We need to be held accountable for how we live after our traumatic event.

I remember many times I couldn't cry sober, so I had to rely on alcohol to release my pain. It helped me deal with triggers and my anxiety. Sometimes I was numb, other times I couldn't handle the pain from the triggers. I needed a 'why' before I could seek help and find change.

Once your mind is determined to let go of fear and confront your triggers, you would find the strength to fight them off. You will learn how to manage them with power. When we wish things turned out differently, it's important to remind ourselves that things have a purpose in life.

I decided to turn my pain into purpose and help the voiceless with my story. You can do the same. When I began to write my memoir, I decided to no longer hide behind the shadows or be a victim. I am a survivor, with a purpose in life. I believe my purpose is to help you find yours.

Keeping your mind busy and active will give you less time to worry about negative thoughts. Self-care is also very important. Take a bubble bath when you feel anxious, listen to some music, re-organize your space, and take a day to relax and watch movies.

Don't allow your past to be your future. Take your life back. Be in charge. Your healing is your responsibility. You are the only one who can do this. Seek help and put in the work to make your healing happen. Never be ashamed of your past, your trauma, or your PTSD. That alone will make you stronger to fight your battles and win.

Always remember, you are not alone. You can use your voice and pain to help yourself and others that are trapped in the PTSD cycle. Be the unbroken. Break off the chains of fear that are holding you back.

You are more than just your story. You are more than your past and your triggers. You deserve to heal. You deserve to live a healthy life. You deserve to be happy.

***"I have heard your prayer and seen your tears; I will heal you." 2 Kings 20-5.***

***"He heals the broken-hearted and binds up their wounds." - Psalm 147-3.***

# Prologue

**Pantea Kalhor**

Thank you so much for reading my book and allowing me to share my insights into PTSD with you. I invited the specialists to help write this book so we can share our real case studies and give you true and practical information about how to recover from PTSD. This information can not be found through Google or in any other books.

We wanted to show you that you're not alone on this journey. Trauma is not the end of the world. We may fall, but we can rise again. Sometimes we need to pause, have a rest, and then start over.

I hope this book has helped you create a vision and plan for your future, a way out of the anxiety, suffering and torture that can come as a consequence of PTSD. May you be armed with enough knowledge to continue with your healing journey.

If you have a story that can inspire others to rebuild their life again, connect with me at http://acechoiceidea.com.

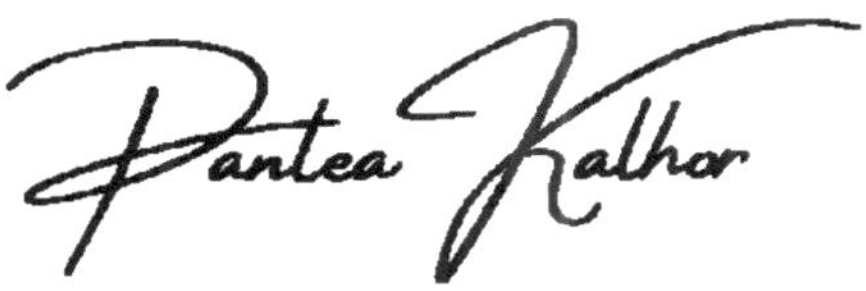

# Part 3: Authors and Contributors

This book is collated and published by Pantea Kalhor and AceChoice Publishing and Branding.

Other Authors: Richard Morden, Linda Hayes Cooper, Maricelly Ramos, Nancy Nance, Roseline Salazar

Other Summit Speakers: Dr Lizette Battaille, Jessica Se Serre Boissonneault, Lise Leblanc, Jeannine L. Rashidi, Dr Achina Stein, Dr Manon Bolliger, Debera Jenson, Jason Coulthard, Debbie Pace

# About the Author, Pantea Kalhor

Pantea Kalhor is 4 x #1 international Best-Selling author of *Rules of Change for the Better* and *Naturally Conceived* and co-author of *Empowering Women to Succeed: Leap.* She's a publisher, podcaster, software engineer, certified PTSD coach, fertility coach, project manager and have a master's degree in information technology.

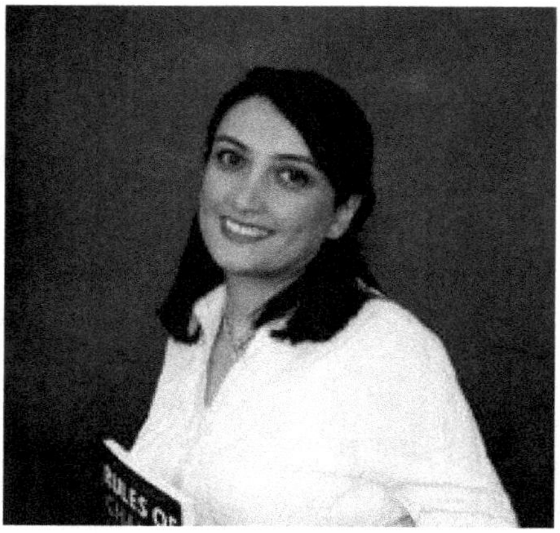

Her mission is to create a bridge between western and eastern medicine. To show how holistic medicine and mind-body connection can help conventional medicine to find the underlying health issues which are usually ignored or left undiscovered. After suffering from PTSD after her car was hijacked and she was threatened by knifepoint, she started her journey of transformation. Years later, she wrote her first book *Rules of Change for The Better* describing her own personal stories of transition. Then she started creating *Transition by Pantea Kalhor,* a podcast with interviews with health care and holistic medicine practitioners, medical doctors, functional medicine practitioners, and PTSD coaches. They share the message of hope and introduce different modalities in Post Trauma recovery.

If you wish to share your message, you can contact me through my website:

http://acechoiceidea.com

**If you are a PTSD Warrior in need of some empowerment, follow me in social media.**

Facebook: https://www.facebook.com/panteakalhorcoach

Instagram: https://www.instagram.com/panteakalhorcoach

YouTube: https://www.youtube.com/c/PanteaKalhorTransition-Channel

Podcast: https://panteakalhor.libsyn.com/

# CONTACT THE EXPERTS

Other Authors: Richard Morden, Linda Hayes Cooper, Maricelly Ramos, Nancy Nance, Roseline Salazar

Other Summit Speakers: Dr Lizette Battaille, Jessica Se Serre Boissonneault, Lise Leblanc, Jeannine L. Rashidi, Dr Achina Stein, Dr Manon Bolliger, Debera Jenson, Jason Coulthard, Debbie Pace

# Nancy Nance, Recovery Coach, Author

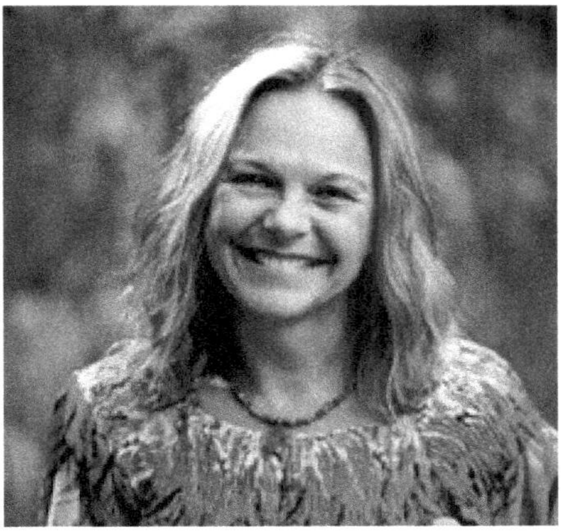

Nancy (Nance) Chaplin is known as Exponential Joy, for she truly has learned to live an exponentially joyful life. Joy is her life. She is the founder and CEO of Exponential Joy. Nancy is a Spiritual Response Therapist (SRT), Reiki Practitioner, Aromatherapist and Light Worker. She uses the many modalities of healing to help clear and balance your energies. Her purpose and passion are to help as many people as possible heal their hears with her *Recover Your joy* Program.

You can access her here:
http://exponentialjoy.com/

Facebook: @exponentialjoy

https://www.youtube.com/channel/UCnY1gf7OFPY0kxYUfAbSajg

# Richard Morden, Certified EFT, Author

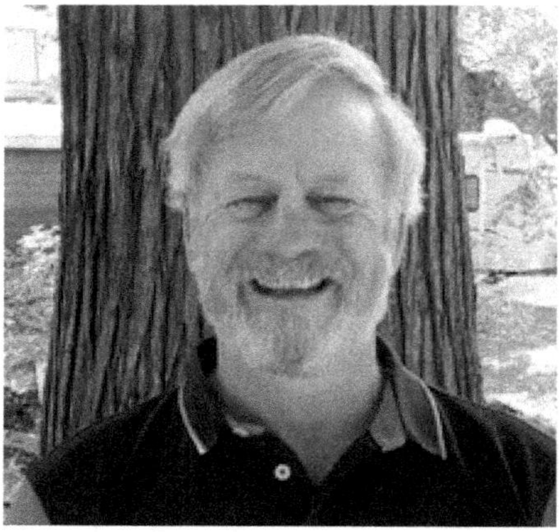

Richard is a Certified EFT (Emotional Freedom Technique) Practitioner, Emotional Success Coach and Body Talk Access Practitioner. Richard uses EFT guided sessions to bring healing to clients who have suffered trauma, PTSD, anxiety, depression, panic attacks, and other deep-rooted issues that often-traditional therapy cannot resolve. Clients are drawn to Richard because of his solution-based approach to overcoming limiting beliefs. He understands the complicated emotions of a breakdown; the new breath that comes with new life, as well as the tension to hold on to pieces of the past. Through virtual or in-person sessions, he teaches the tools of self-care to empower clients. Guided self-help techniques in EFT can restore clarity and purpose and remove personal trauma that hides in the protected vaults of our minds. Richard's own vulnerability helps him provide a practice where safe progress is balanced with a tender approach to remove the barriers and heaviness that surrounds personal trauma.
www.qapproach.com

https://www.facebook.com/LifeTransititionCoachRichardMorden

https://www.linkedin.com/in/richard-morden/

# Linda Hayes Cooper, Early Parenting Therapist, Author

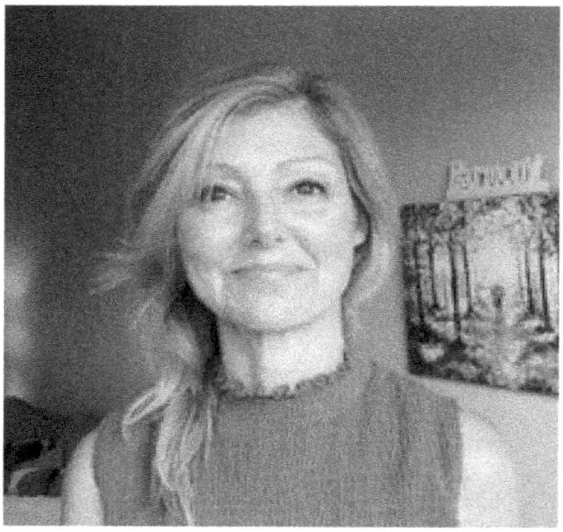

Linda Hayes-Cooper is an Early Parenting Therapist, Clinical Psychologist helping new and expectant parents move from WORRIERS to WARRIORS so they can live the family life of their dreams. She is the founder of *Calm Emotional Presence* that cultivates your 'designer footprint' fast tracking to mental health and wellbeing. She has a particular interest in the mental health of infants, toddlers and pre-schoolers. Linda has over 25-years of training and experience working with young families as a psychologist, midwife, baby whisperer, and breastfeeding consultant. She is the author of her upcoming book *Footprints* – bringing awareness of trans-generational patterns and implementations that cultivate healthier attachment relationships in young families. Linda has been featured in The Sydney Morning Herald, Offspring Parenting magazine, North Sydney Times, and Angus Cameron's Handbook of Pediatric Dentistry (2nd, 3rd & 4th Ed.) Linda has completed M.Psyc

Clinical, B.Psyc Honors, B.Health Sci - Nursing, Midwifery Certificate, Child & Family Health certificate. She is trained in psychological techniques such as NLP, CBT, ACT, MiCBT, Mindfulness, DMM Attachment model, and various parenting programs such as COS, WWW, CARE-INDEX for infants and toddlers. www.lindacep.com
Instagram and Facebook: @lindahayestherapy

# Roseline Salazar, Retired Air Force Military Officer, PTSD Coach, Author

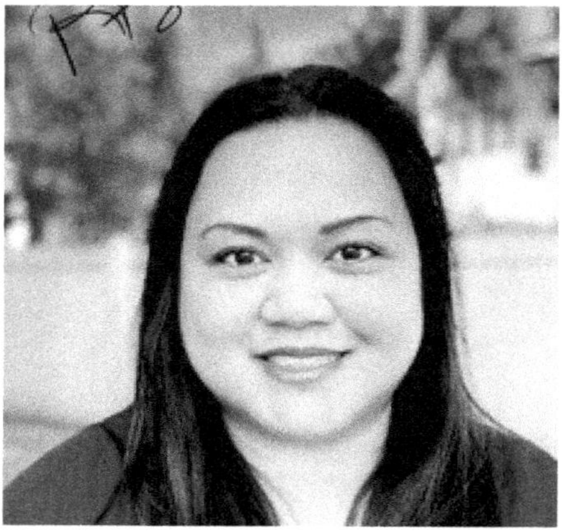

Roseline F. Pagala Salazar, prior Air Force Major, was born and raised in Honolulu, Hawaii. As a child, she was inspired to join the military by her two older brothers, who were in the Hawaii Army National Guard. About a year after her father's death in 1995, she joined the U.S. Air Force to have a better life and provide for her immediate family back home. Upon retiring in March 2012, she enjoyed raising her two children and earned her degree in paralegal studies. Rosaline holds a B.S. in information systems management from the University of Maryland University College, an M.S. in management with a concentration in human resources from Troy University, an A.S. in paralegal studies from the Kapiolani Community College, and an A.S. in transportation from the Community College of the Air Force. She currently resides in Hawaii with her two children, Zoe and Zachary, along with the rest of her family. She is also a combat veteran, just started her mental

health coaching business and looking forward to her new journey as an author.
http://www.roselinesalazar.com

https://www.instagram.com/roselinefsalazar/

# Maricelly Ramnos, Certified Life Coach, Author

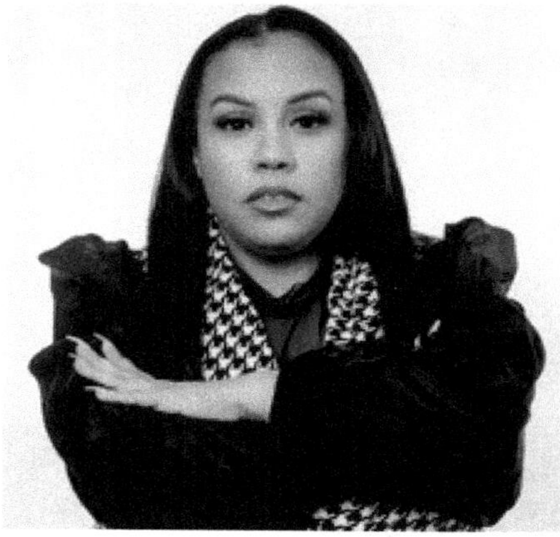

Maricelly is a domestic violence survivor who was diagnosed with PTSD from the trauma of her relationships. As a result, she has had to identify what her triggers are and learn how to cope with them and heal. People walking behind her, too close to her, looking at her for too long, or touching her, are just some of the triggers she has suffered from. But Maricelly has learned coping mechanisms like using her breathing skills to control her emotions and speaking positive affirmations out loud so her brain can hear and adjust accordingly. She is now an author, certified life coach, and entrepreneur. Maricelly also helps women reconnect with themselves after they escape the cycle of abuse. http://www.MaricellyRamos.com

Instagram: Maricelly_Ramos

Facebook: Maricelly Ramos

# Erin Chandler, intuitive guide and psychic medium, Contributor

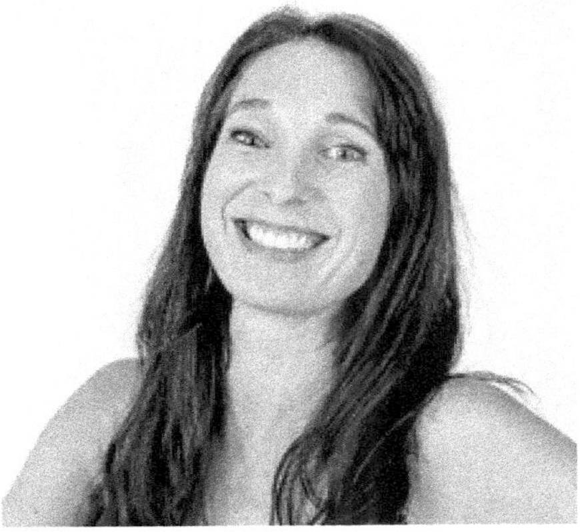

Erin Chandler is an Intuitive grief coach, author, speaker and creator of the *'Grieve, Release and Connect'* program. As a bereaved parent and psychic medium, Erin accesses intuitive information and guidance of the highest levels to facilitate healing on multiple levels of trauma. Going one step further, she teaches others how to tap into their own spiritual guidance for the ultimate healing and transformation of grief, loss, and trauma. Chandler has dedicated her life to helping others overcome trauma and living a full and excited life again. As an Amazon best-selling author of *'Love you Ava Baby'* and *'The Spirit Connection'*, she shares the highs and lows of trauma, grief and loss, as well as the spiritual guidance and tools she used to overcome and transform her life with passion and purpose.
https://www.erinchandler.com/

# Dr. Lizette Bataille, Medical Director, Contributor

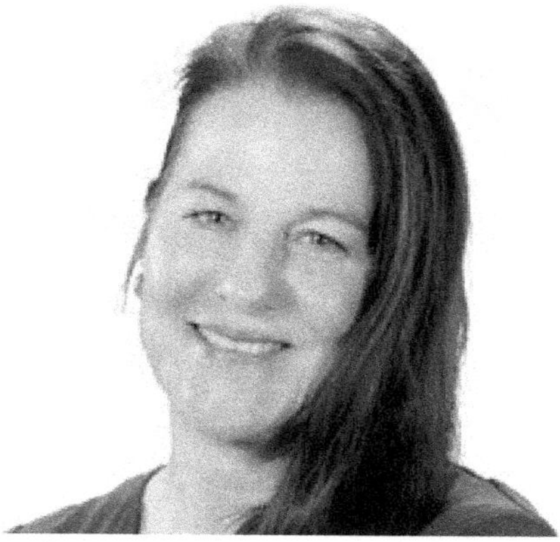

Dr. Liz knows that hope will get you back to a life you love again. From experiencing loss to sexual abuse, addiction, and suicidal ideation, Dr. Liz knows trauma, abuse, and grief. Throughout her work with professionals and a 12-step program, she survived her traumas and found the strength to move forward with hope. Her purpose drives her desire to help others find peace and joy in their life after surviving trauma. At the ARISE! Mind, Body, Spirit Healing Institute, Dr. Liz provides holistic healing strategies, education, and practices to help you thrive beyond trauma, abuse, addiction, or suicidal ideation. Her healing exercises awaken the mind, body, and spirit to a new joy in life. With 30-years in the medical field, Dr. Liz is well educated in the workings of the human body and the healing practices that get things back on track. She's an international best-selling author with her first

nonfiction book, *Life Launch - Surviving the Storms of Physical and Sexual Abuse, Book One.*
http://www.drlizlifelaunch.com

https://www.instagram.com/drlizlifelaunch/

https://www.facebook.com/drlizlifelaunch

# Jessica De Serre Boissonneault, Flight Attendant, Contributor

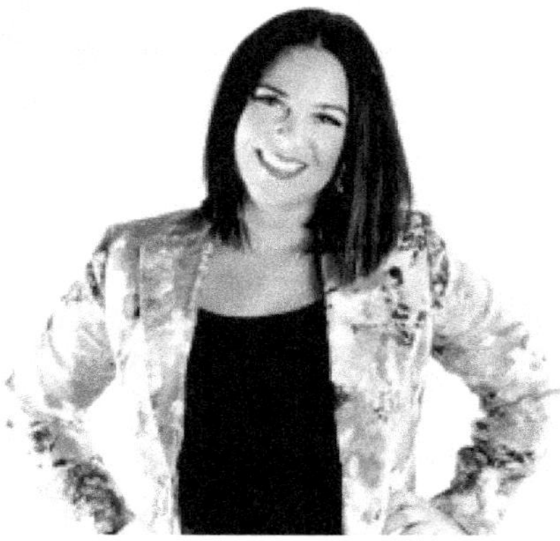

From small-town girl to global inspiration, Jessica has always been known for her positivity and bubbliness! She studied Sociology to follow her passion for helping others and is certified in NLP. She is a lifetime learner and has personal growth as an integral part of her daily routine. Following her mission of supporting women, Jessica started her own podcast show and founded the *Women Empowerment Wednesday Show.* She is the founder of the *Take Flight Coaching Academy,* serving you as Your Empowerment Agent. She was nominated for Top 50 Most Influential Women in the VIP Global Magazine in the United States and is an award-winning author with two International-Best-Selling Books. Her third book will book was launched in June 2021, called *I am a Flight Attendant and that is my Superpower.* Jessica's real transformation began in 2013 when she made the crucial decision to escape an abusive marriage and start her journey as a single mother. She

leaned on her power, passion, and unbending positivity to transform herself, and in doing so, she learned how to elevate women just like her. Jessica is about to launch her group coaching program to elevate women to live a purposeful and powerful life. Her motto is:
***"We rise by lifting each other!"***

She is dedicated to sharing her contagious energy with everyone fortunate enough to cross her path.

Instagram: @ms.jessicadsb

Facebook: Jessica De Serre Boissonneault

# Lise Leblanc - Registered psychotherapist, Contributor

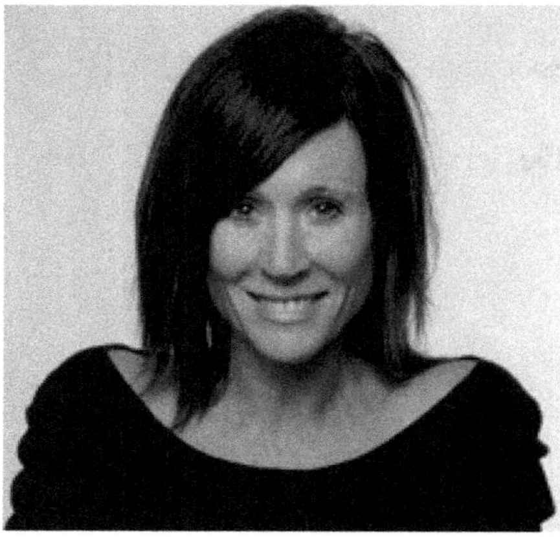

As a registered psychotherapist with over 20-years of experience working in therapeutic, educational, and leadership roles, Lise Leblanc has seen first-hand the profound impact traumatic experiences can have on a person's life. Lise has a bachelor's degree in psychology and a master's degree in educational leadership, as well as many clinical certifications. However, most of her knowledge does not come from books. It comes from overcoming her own traumatic experiences and personal challenges and working with hundreds of clients to help them overcome theirs. Lise continues to work in private practice, specializing in anxiety, depression, grief, and trauma. She uses the same holistic and eclectic approach that helped her on own healing journey. Along with her PTSD Workbook, her mission in writing her PTSD Guide is to give readers the knowledge, insight, and strategies to clear out the fear, shame, and trauma that is keeping them in a painful cycle of suffering.

Lise's first book, *Conscious Caregiving Guide,* and second book, *Conscious Grief and Loss Guide,* are also currently available.
https://liseleblanc.ca

https://www.facebook.com/liseleblancnextchapterpress

Instagram: @liseleblanc100

# Jeannine L. Rashidi, health & wellness practitioner

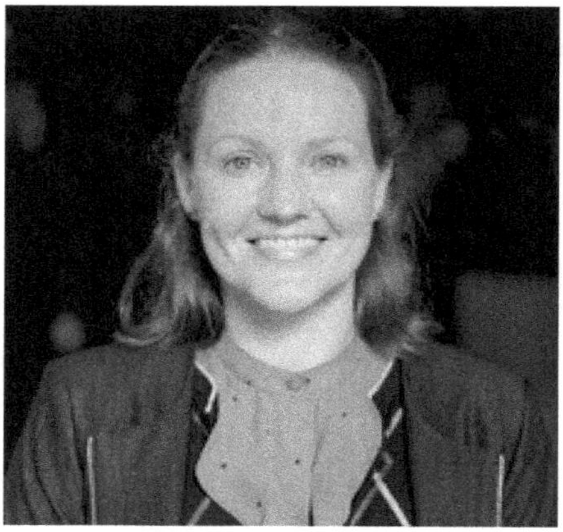

Jeannine Rashidi is a highly qualified health and wellness practitioner. She opened her Goodbye Tension practice in 2003, focused on alleviating the core of physical, digestive, emotional, and mental tension. Her commitment to empower and inspire her clients towards awakening the healer within has been a passion for the last 18-years. She has experience healing 25-years of trauma & PTSD, and her book *Abundance Beyond Trauma* is helpful for anyone who has experienced Trauma, PTSD, and other adverse life experiences. Her book is an excellent resource for all health and wellness practitioners and doctors.

It teaches on understanding the mind and the process that guides clients and patients towards healing themselves. Jeannine is also an Ayurvedic Practitioner currently enrolled in the Ayurvedic Doctorate program at Kerala Ayurveda Academy. She has apprenticed under Dr. Jayarajan Kodikannath since 2016, traveled to Kerala to experience the roots of Ayurveda, and is an ongoing Samskritam (Sanskrit) student, so she is able to study the source Ayurvedic books directly. Jeannine is a devoted wife, mother, and recent grandmother.

Instagram, Facebook: @ GoodbyeTension,
https://www.goodbyetension.com

# Dr Achina Stein, DO, DFAPA, FACN, ABIHM, IFMCP, Contributor

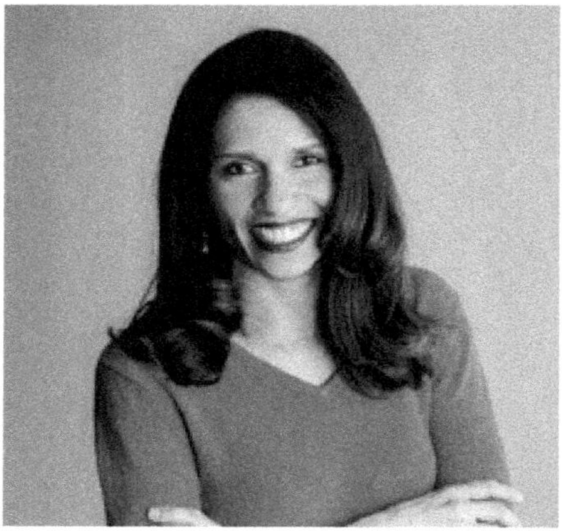

Achina P. Stein DO, DFAPA, FACN, ABIHM, IFMCP Functional Mind, LLC, Co-owner is an osteopathic physician (DO) who graduated from Rowan University School of Osteopathic Medicine in 1990. She has been in practice as a board-certified psychiatrist for 25 plus years. Her osteopathic roots set her apart from the conventional psychiatrists because of her use of osteopathic philosophy and the bio-psycho-social treatment approach. She trained in psychodynamic psychotherapy and CBT and does psychotherapy with several people with underlying trauma issues, specifically mood and dissociative disorders. She has a wealth of experience working with the prison population, community mental health center, the chronic mental health population, and geriatric psychiatry inpatients. Her book, *What If It's NOT Depression? Your Guide to Answers and Solutions,* launched in February 2020 and became an International Bestseller in 3 categories on Amazon Kindle. Dr.

Achina Stein is also author of *What If It's NOT Depression? Your Guide to Finding Answers and Solutions.* She has a busy private practice called Functional Mind LLC in Riverside, RI.
www.achinasteindo.com

Facebook: @AchinaSteinD, Instagram: @dr.achinstein

# Dr. Manon Bolliger, ND, Founder of Bowen Therapy, Contributor

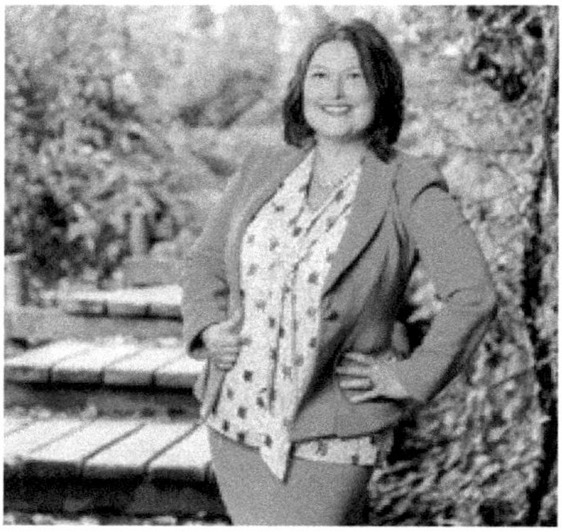

As a Naturopathic Medical Doctor and CEO of Bowen College, where she has trained over 2500 healthcare practitioners, Dr. M (Manon) Bolliger helps people take ownership of their choices in health. She is launching a Global Health Initiative based on collaboration and consolidation of complementary health practices for both impact and value. The best-selling author of '*What Patients Don't Say if Doctors Don't Ask*', her expertise is in chronic physical and emotional pain, trauma, and shifting people to a mindset focused on "health-nosis" and not a "dia-gnosis". While overcoming stage 4 CA (cancer and carcinoma) without pharmaceutical or a hysterectomy, she discovered that we are accustomed to thinking that conflict resolution is mediated externally. But when it comes to health, it is an internal process. She has pioneered the '*A Healer in Every Household*' Movement embracing the body's capacity to heal and the choice to govern how we live our lives. Her new book, '*A Healer in Every Household: Looking Beyond Your Symptoms*', was launched in September 2020. She has spoken on international stages like JTFoxx's Money, Health and Business, TEDx talk in Las Vegas, is the host of *The Healer's Cafe* podcast and has appeared on ABC, CTV and NBC, https://www.bowencollege.com/

www.rebootyourbody.info

# Debera Jensen, Rapid Relief Energy Healer, Contributor

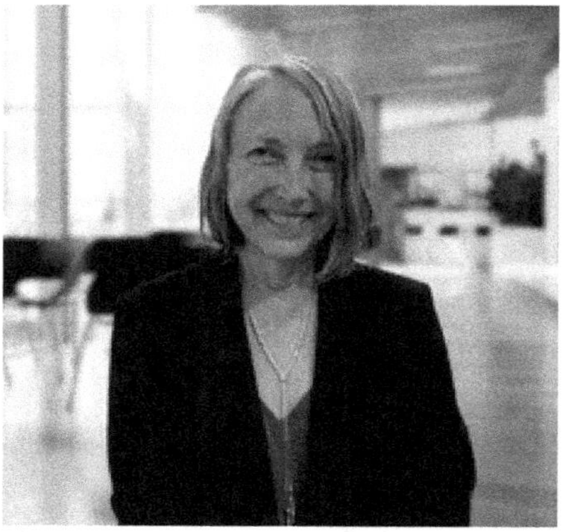

Debera Jensen is a Rapid Relief Energy/Mindset and Belief Healer who was in a horrific accident many years ago from which she was not expected to recover. She had a severe concussion and spinal injuries which caused unrelenting pain. Debera eventually found her way out of those injuries which, oddly enough, highlighted her earlier childhood traumas. She was finally able to heal and now she enjoys a very joyous life. She opened an Alternative Center where she now helps people to leave behind the trauma, concussions, and stress. She believes that when a business owner releases the trauma, their business grows and are much more focused and successful.
Quantum Entrepreneurs Making the Impossible Possible Facebook group

https://www.facebook.com/groups/881809652576794

# Jason Coulthard, Former Crime Enforcement Detective, Contributor

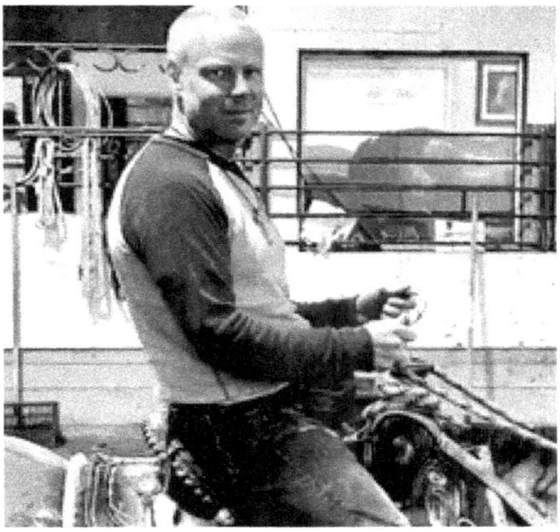

Former Homicide and International Organized Crime Enforcement Detective Jason Coulthard worked with the Toronto Police Service for 21 years. As a result of this and unresolved childhood issues, he ended up with several Operational Stress Injuries that have been healed outside of our currently insurable system in Canada. As part of his journey of healing that started in December 2017, he had a supernatural experience after attending a healing retreat. After he returned, he miraculously healed himself from all of my physical signs, symptoms, syndromes and diseases previously experienced and no longer needs medication. However, the psychiatrists he saw, did not believe this. Due to his behaviour, he was committed under the mental health act for 21-days. He and many others from across Canada are coming together to build the first New Hope Field of Dreams - Family Revival Retreat. Then they plan to do that worldwide. Their goal is to change

the way the healthcare system works, specifically the area of mental health. They are going to present the problem, provide solutions, and promote these solutions.
www.newhopefieldofdreams.ca

# Debbie Pace, intuitive inner freedom coach, Contributor

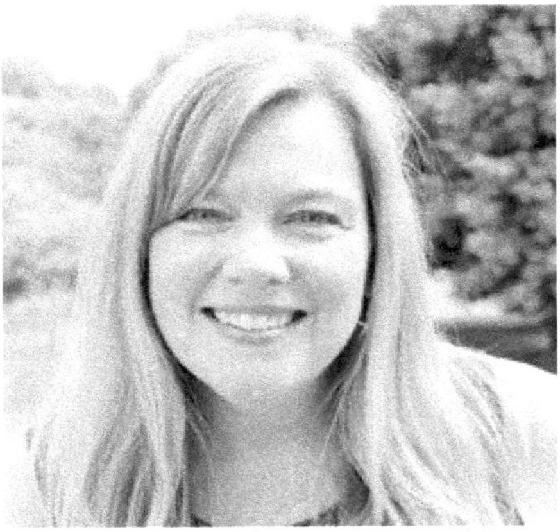

Debbie Pace is an inspirational leader, certified Quantum Flow practitioner, Reiki master, author of *The Journal to Freedom,* an intuitive inner freedom coach and host of *The Show Up!* Podcast. She is also a triathlete and a firewalker, 4x and counting. She is a former U.S. Navy Journalist with nearly three decades of award-winning military and commercial broadcast experience.

Debbie's experience is also with radio and TV news anchoring, reporting online news. Editing, writing, and producing. She even has some country music DJ'ing. Debbie brings an MBA, NLP, Sound Healing, Akashic Record Clearing, and many other trainings to coach powerhouse clients to overcome any and EVERY obstacle, keeping them from fully stepping into a life of freedom and connecting with the power and purity of their soul.

Facebook: https://www.facebook.com/DebbiePaceGlobal

Instagram: https://www.instagram.com/debbiepaceglobal/

Podcast: https://www.theshowupshow.com/

# References


1. ^ Intuitive healer, psychic medium, author, and teacher, www.erinchandler.com
2. ^ Rules of Change for The Better: Real stories and your guide to tune-up your mood and transform your life to reach your biggest dreams, https://www.amazon.com/dp/B07L3D6XT1
3. ^ Naturally Conceived: How to Get Pregnant, Explain Unexplained Infertility, and Prevent Miscarriages By Unleashing Your Reproductive https://www.amazon.com/dp/B08FTJNR57/
4. ^ https://www.amazon.com/dp/B07L3D6XT1
5. ^ Transition by Pantea Kalhor (libsyn.com)
6. ^ Hidden Pandemic': 1 million Children Worldwide Lost A Parent To Covid, Study Finds, https://tinyurl.com/Forbes-Covid-Loss
7. ^ https://youtu.be/gn6nfo7a_cg
8. ^ https://www.amazon.com/dp/B08FTJNR57/
9. ^ https://www.researchgate.net/publication/284277270_Prenatal_Bonding_Bindungsanalyse_by_Raffai_-_An_Introduction
10. ^ https://www.amazon.com/dp/B07L3D6XT1/
11. ^ Life Launch: Surviving the Storms of Physical and Sexual Abuse: https://www.amazon.com/dp/B07V3N3YL5
12. ^ Ayurveda and Traditional Chinese Medicine: A Comparative Overview, https://www.ncbi.nlm.nih.gov/pmc/articles/PMC1297513/
13. ^ Abundance Beyond Trauma: Discovering Your Courage for Change and Commitment to Yourself: Rashidi, Jeannine L,

Purdin, Wayne, Kodikannath, Jayarajan: 9781736664803: Amazon.com: Books

14. ^ Gut-Brain Connection: Microbiome, Gut Barrier, and Environmental Sensors, https://www.ncbi.nlm.nih.gov/pmc/articles/PMC8263213/
15. ^ The Action Guide to Healing from Childhood Trauma can help. www.thetraumahealingcoach.com
16. ^ Aging Magnificently and Powerfully, Dr Defne Nayman, Green Healing Show, https://youtu.be/QzyvjP-GPxg
17. ^ You, Me & PTSD-The Intruder in My Marriage, Sajel Bellon, PTSD Self-Healing Show, https://youtu.be/UuCce4pr1F4
18. ^ Project Infinity saw police seize $79M worth of drugs: https://www.cbc.ca/news/canada/toronto/project-infinity-saw-police-seize-79m-worth-of-drugs-1.1868159
19. ^ Adverse Childhood Experiences (ACEs): https://www.cdc.gov/violenceprevention/aces/index.html
20. ^ Linda Hayes Website: www.lindacep.com
21. ^ PTSD: Learn about symptoms and treatment | Mental Health | communityhealthmagazine.com

CPSIA information can be obtained
at www.ICGtesting.com
Printed in the USA
LVHW080513030322
712522LV00004B/124

9 781778 035128